OTOPLASTY
Aesthetic and Reconstructive Techniques

Springer
*New York
Berlin
Heidelberg
Barcelona
Budapest
Hong Kong
London
Milan
Paris
Santa Clara
Singapore
Tokyo*

OTOPLASTY
Aesthetic and Reconstructive Techniques

Jack Davis, M.D.

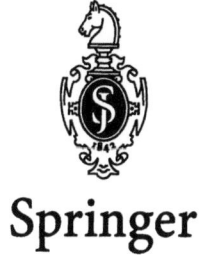

Springer

Jack Davis, MD
Buenos Aires University
Department of Plastic Surgery
Gelly 3460
1425 Buenos Aires
Argentina
011.5401.801.6479 (phone/fax)

Library of Congress Cataloging-in-Publication Data
Davis, Jack, 1918–
　Otoplasty: aesthetic and reconstructive techniques/Jack Davis.—2nd ed.
　　p. cm.
　Rev. ed. of: Aesthetic and reconstructive otoplasty/Jack Davis.
c 1987.
　Includes bibliographical references and index.
　　ISBN-13: 978-1-4612-7484-1　　　e-ISBN-13: 978-1-4612-2276-7
　DOI: 10.1007/978-1-4612-2276-7

　　1. Otoplasty.　I. Davis, Jack, 1918–　Aesthetic and
reconstructive otoplasty.　II. Title.
　　[DNLM: 1. Ear, External—surgery.　2. Surgery, Plastic—methods.
WV 220 D262o 1997]
RF127.D38　1997
617.8′0592—dc20
DNLM/DLC
for Library of Congress　　　　　　　　　　　　　　　　　　　96-35161
　　　　　　　　　　　　　　　　　　　　　　　　　　　　　　　　CIP

Printed on acid-free paper.

©1997 Springer-Verlag New York Inc.
Softcover reprint of the hardcover 1st edition 1997

All rights reserved. This work may not be translated or copied in whole or in part without the written permission of the publisher (Springer-Verlag New York, Inc., 175 Fifth Avenue, New York, NY 10010. USA), except for brief excerpts in connection with reviews or scholarly analysis. Use in connection with any form of information and retrieval, electronic adaptation, computer software, or by similar or dissimilar methodology now known or hereafter developed is forbidden.
The use of general descriptive names, trade names, trademarks, etc., in this publication, even if the former are not especially identified, is not to be taken as a sign that such names, as understood by the Trade Marks and Merchandise Marks Act, may accordingly be used freely by anyone.
While the advice and information in this book are believed to be true and accurate at the date of going to press, neither the authors nor the editors nor the publisher can accept any legal responsibility for any errors or omissions that may be made. The publisher makes no warranty, express or implied, with respect to the material contained herein.

Typeset by University Graphics, Inc., York, PA.

9 8 7 6 5 4 3 2 1

Contents

Foreword *vii*
Acknowledgments *xi*

1 The Patient *1*
Ear Inferiority Complex   *2*

2 Aesthetic Otoplasty *3*
Secondary Otoplasty   *3*
Conchal Flap   *9*
Cryptotia and Satyr Ear   *10*
Trauma   *14*
Healing Potential   *20*
Keloids   *20*
Test for Measurement of Delicacy   *23*

3 Moderate Microtia and Partial Atresia *24*
Embryology of the External Ear   *24*
Analysis of Branchial Apparatus Concepts   *25*
Microtia and Auricular Atresia   *31*
Otologic Criteria   *33*
Should Unilateral Atresis be Operated On?   *33*
Auricular Atresia   *34*
Canal   *35*
Partial Atresia Syndromes   *36*

4 The Cartilage *43*
Basic Considerations   *44*
Nutrition   *44*
Varieties   *45*
Histogenesis, Growth, and Regeneration   *46*
Investigation   *46*
Auricular Functional Properties   *54*
Pinna–Partial Canal Syndrome   *58*
Moderate Microtia and Total Atresia   *63*

5 Severe Microtia and Radical Auriculoplasty *66*
Unilateral Microtia   *67*
Auricular Integument   *68*
Davis Tests   *71*
Helical Sulcus   *72*
Total Auricular Atresia   *86*
Surgery   *88*
Results   *98*
Secondary Strictures   *99*

6 Bilateral Microtia and Atresia *101*

Bilateral Atresia *103*

Upper Nubbin *104*

Framework *104*

Severe Microtia Repaired Only with Microtial Cartilage of the Same Side *107*

7 Hemifacial Microsomia *111*

Measure of Results *114*

8 Conclusion *115*

Bibliography *116*

Index *133*

Foreword

In keeping with my longstanding interest in the surgical corrrection of external ear deformities, I have followed Jack Davis' contributions to this challenging type of reconstructive and aesthetic plastic surgery since I read his first article in 1951. As a longtime good friend of Jack in our roles as editors of the journal, *Aesthetic Plastic Surgery,* and as past presidents of the International Society of Aesthetic Plastic Surgery (ISAPS), I have kept up-to-date in reading his numerous accomplishments in external ear surgery for these past 46 years.

The reader might find it reassuring to learn that in this period of $4\frac{1}{2}$ decades, Jack Davis has contributed to our specialty 42 separate articles, lectures, discussions, chapters, and other items describing external ear surgery. In 1978 in our journal, *Aesthetic Plastic Surgery,* he presented an excellent review article on "History of the Aesthetic Surgery of the Ear," which was co-authored with the assistance of Horacio H. Hernandez. This same subject was also presented in 1985 in a chapter in an ISAPS book devoted to the "The Creation of Aesthetic Plastic Surgery." Even more importantly, and historically, Davis gave us his *opus magnum* publication in 1987, *Aesthetic and Reconstructive Otoplasty,* which covered almost every conceivable aspect of these types of surgery in its 581 pages.

With his outstanding ability as a very thorough historian, his 1987 book had 1,711 references. In this current 1997 volume there are an additional 567 references to these very valuable combined bibliographies. Since he first started publishing medical articles in English and Spanish, lecturing in both languages, and contributing chapters and discussions to numerous books internationally, one is not surprised to find that since 1951 Davis has published 9 otoplasty articles in English, 6 in Spanish, 13 otoplasty chapters in English books, 4 chapters in Spanish books, 5 lectures at international symposia in English, and 5 lectures in Spanish. It should not surprise the reader, that in his early and mid-career as a plastic and reconstructive surgeon, Davis has been a very fine hand surgeon as well. He was probably the first in the Southern Hemisphere to report 3 successful cases of toe-to-hand transfers in 1964 in an article that contained a wealth of very accurate historical information about this fascinating operation, the first successful operation being performed by Nicoladoni of Graz, Austria in 1900.

In considering all of Davis' valuable contributions to surgery of the external ear, he remains one of the few continually interested members and experts of that small group of plastic surgeons who have, throughout the whole world, been noted for their efforts in this field, including Avelar, Barinka, Brent, Fukuda, Furnas, Mustarde, Nagata, Oulie, Senechal, Tanzer, and a few others. For those of us who know Jack Davis personally, within a few minutes of his stimulating conversation, tinged with his fine British accent, it becomes quickly apparent that his enthusiasm is limitless, especially when he speaks of his favorite subject, the reconstructive and aesthetic surgery of the ear. Davis comes from an English heritage, and by working at the British Hospial in Buenos Aires his Argentinean citizenship makes him essentially a Renaissance man of two worlds—not only of the English-speaking world with its wonderful and expansive contributions to the whole field of plastic, reconstructive, and aesthetic surgery, but of the Spanish and Portuguese-speaking medical world as well, with whose vast literature he is extremely familiar and cites again and again in the bibliography of this current "updated volume."

His pioneering book in 1987 has been expanded in this latest volume in a slightly different medium and presented as an "update." The illustrations and drawings in the volume were made once again by Davis himself. A mere glance at its table of contents shows us that the scope of his present interest ranges far afield, evidenced by several of the chapters cited being devoted to Secondary Otoplasty, Conchal Floor Composite Flap, Traumatic Avulsion, the Problem of Keloids, Auditory Canal and Partial Atresia, Histogenesis and Growth of Ear Cartilage, Expansion Chondrotomy, Stereotaxic Surgery for Total Atresia, Late Revision, Secondary Strictures, and Hemifacial Microsomia. In this "updated volume," Davis shows us a modest number of highly selective problems that have often made solutions very difficult in previous years for most of the very experienced surgeons who are considered some of the "masters" in the field.

This smaller "update" volume is not as comprehensive in its overall aspects as Davis' 1987 book and was not intended to be. But as a critical "update," it is a fascinating description by the author of very specific problems in a dozen or more highly individualized cases that have proven many times in the recent past to be challenges not always met with or resolved by the then available techniques—not only in reconstructive but aesthetic surgery of external ear problems as well.

In this latest book, Davis treats us to his own personal and very artistic approach to taking on these difficult cases and narrates for us, in a step-by-step teaching fashion, the philosophy and planning behind his repair and how it was accomplished. These "updated" techniques and cases are accompanied by a large number of excellent pre- and post-operative photographs that show us the gradual step-by-step progress of the repair of these deformities. It seems appropriate to emphasize that in his final conclusion to this "update," Davis has come to a rather profound summary of his ideas when he states that, "attempting to analyze and establish a breakdown of my 92 completed ear reconstructions with rib cartilage and 352 with ear cartilage is rather pointless. There are too many variables for the results to be mathematically significant."

The reader can see, therefore, that both of these books, the 1987 volume and this 1997 "update" volume, represent the lifetime experience of a very talented, very observant, and truly compassionate plastic, reconstructive, and aesthetic surgeon.

Blair O. Rogers, M.D., F.A.C.S.
Professor of Clinical Surgery (Plastic Surgery)
New York University Medical Center
Editor-in-Chief, *Aesthetic Plastic Surgery*

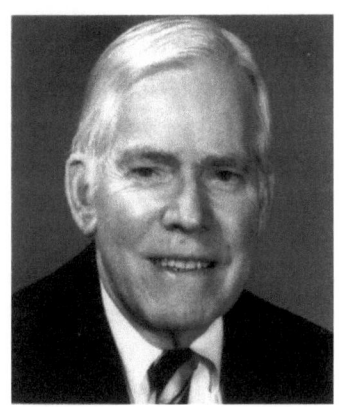

My friends,

My mother used to say: *"Nothing stands still. You go forward or you go back."* I probably agree with her about otoplasty. A book's value is not to applaud the author, but to contribute knowledge, by learning what went well, what did not, and why, and the measure of results. Very gracious book reviews have labelled *Aesthetic and Reconstructive Otoplasty* (1987) a *"Bible"* on the subject. But now, recent advances make this update timely and indicated. The 1987 text remains basic.

A spark of understanding has pierced the clouds of habit, dogmatic repetition, customary thought, and procedure. The spark grew, and something new was born. A way of thinking broke through, that had to be proven by putting it to the test. Accepted assertions were revised, reviewed, differently interpreted, and changed. The horizon cleared. The challenge has been not only to make an ear look human, but be human. It was a new dimension. It has been done.

The starting point was embryologic investigation and reconsideration. The test has been tissue research in the laboratory. The review has been learning the value of auricular multifunction, and knowing the syndrome to be one unit.

This paved the way. Surgical application of these findings proved true in practice. New methods were created and refined, and took shape with multidisciplinary teamwork. Desired results were obtained. They can now be published.

This millennium is closing as a milestone in otoplasty. A new era is dawning.

J. D.

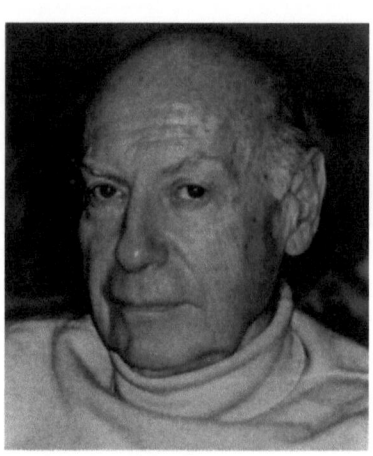

The author

Acknowledgments

This book is produced by a host of anonymous contributors. I want to thank the members of the British Hospital, French Hospital, German Hospital, Spanish Hospital, Castex Hospital, Vicente Lopez Hospital, Durand Hospital, Clínicas University Hospital, and Mater Dei Clinic, all of Buenos Aires, for their backing and help.

Prize-winning surgeon Gustavo Grgicevic is worthy of special mention for his work in anatomy and pathologic research.

I am again indebted to Blair Rogers for his very kind foreword.

My gratitude to the staff of Springer-Verlag for a superb effort in a short period of time to get this information to the reader. And to the reader, with the hope that through him or her the patients will be better served, because they are precisely the most important part of this book.

For allowing reproduction of their work, my special recognition is due to Butterworth and Co., Churchill-Livingstone Inc., Elsevier Biomedical Press, Excerpta Medica, Little, Brown and Co., Piccin Nova Libreria, W.B. Saunders Co., and Springer-Verlag.

It is the wish of the author that it be known that the following awards have been granted to contributers of this book:

FIRST PRIZE to Gustavo Grgcevic at the Anatomy Association Congress, Argentina, 1992, for "Embriología de los Arcos Branquiales",

FIRST PRIZE to Gustavo Grgcevic at the Annual Congress for Plastic and Reconstructive Surgery, Argentina, 1992 for "Secturización de la Oreja" (RESEARCH),

FIRST PRIZE to Gustavo Grgcevic at the Annual Congress for Plastic and Reconstructive Surgery, Argentina, 1993 for "Conceptualización del Primer y Segundo Arco Branquial" (RESEARCH),

FIRST PRIZE to Jack Davis, Oscar Candás, Manuel Martinez, José Rosler and Gustavo Grgcevic for the British Hospital, Buenos Aires, 150 year ANNIVERSARY, 1995, for "Cirugía Estereotáxica para el tallado del Neo-Conducto Auditivo Externo en las Microtias",

FIRST PRIZE to Jack Davis and Gustavo Grgcevic at the Annual Congress for Plastic and Reconstructive Surgery, Argentina, 1996, for "Sindrome Morfo-Auricular del 6° mes: Conceptualización Ontofunctional" (RESEARCH).

1 The Patient

The worst error in otoplasty is to be only a surgical carpenter, forgetting that the most important factor is the patient.

I often remember my medical mentor, Jorge Mulcahy. As I laid flowers on the simple grass patch he had wished as a grave, and felt his gentle smile upon me, I tried to say, "Thank you for so much. So, so much."

I recall an exceptionally pretty nurse, who had been bitten by a dog, which lacerated her ear and cheek. Our local Pasteur Institute supplied rabies serum, and the dog was caged under observation. Vaccination then consisted of 40 injections, one a day. After the fifth she reacted with generalized allergic erythema, and the next day she nearly died, suffocated with edema of Quincke. Mulcahy came and we examined her. He concluded that we could continue the vaccinations daily under 5 hours of general anesthesia. She completed the series and survived. Her ear and face were fine. The dog died of rabies.

I was called late one night by an emergency ward chief. "Come now," he insisted. When I arrived he told me that a patient kept asking for me, and he thought I was her lover and took me at once to see her. She had thrown herself under a subway train, and as her body rotated between the wheels, they cut off both arms and both legs. I asked to see them, and was shown a mass of useless destroyed flesh wrapped up in a newspaper. She held me with her eyes, fixed me with a vise of vision, and desperately demanded, "Doctor, kill me." She was wheeled into surgery.

She was not my lover, but had been a successful modern classical dancer, and I had done a moderate mastoplasty upon her 3 weeks before. The early surgical result was good. She then, however, argued with her father and attempted suicide. During my consultation with Mulcahy he was adamant: "If she wants to live, we will help her to live, and if she wants to die, we will help her to die. Bring her right into our hospital and I will pay the bill." And so it was that I did successive reconstruction on her ears, face, and amputations, and during them she confided that she had changed her mind during her plunge.

She was discharged from the hospital 3 months later and commenced reeducation. In a few months she telephoned me when she won a Ping-Pong tournament with adapted prostheses, progressed to set up a successful business, and married a man younger than herself. I have seen her and

Figure 1

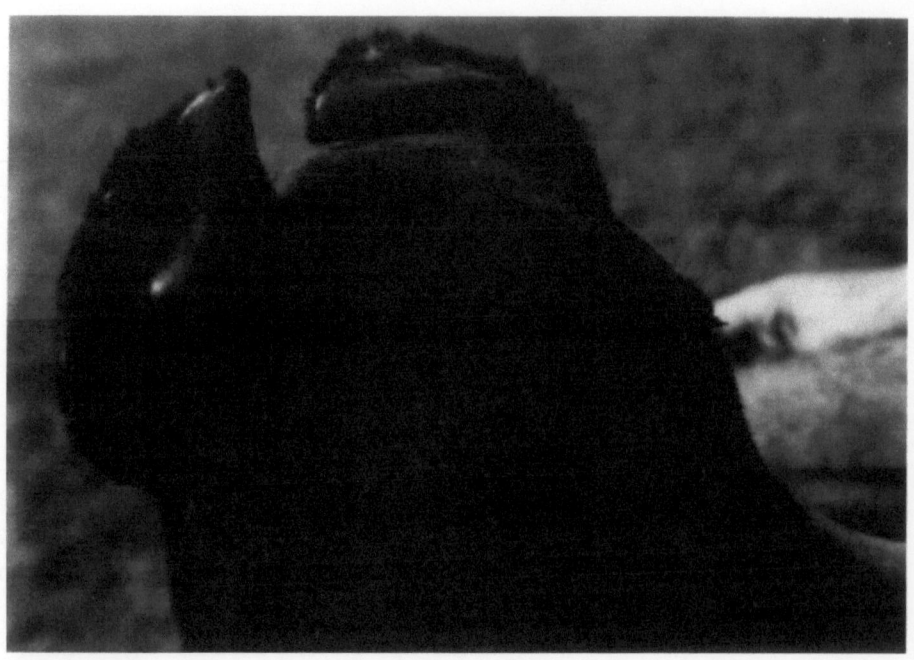

her husband through the years; they are quite inseparable and he tells me, "It is marvelous just being close to her." The combined effort had helped build her up from the ashes. Part of auriculoplasty? Yes, it is part of ear reconstruction.

Ear Inferiority Complex

In contrast to psychoanalysts, I like to think of complexes in a simple way.

Gaucho was a 9-month-old Doberman, but he had a complex. When attentive or excited his ears wrapped over his head instead of pointing straight up (Fig. 1). Everyone laughed at him. He was quite conscious of the ridicule, so he ran away and hid in corners. His owner needed a good watchdog to guard his suburban home, and he had decided that Gaucho should be sacrificed.

He was such a lovely dog that I arranged for his reconstruction. My anesthetist put him to sleep on the garage table. I excised the offending superior auricular muscles, shaped and taped his ears, and just finished the second side when he started to wake up. The result was quite successful, and he became an excellent watchdog with no complex at all.

Somatopsychic? Absolutely.

2 Aesthetic Otoplasty

A few cases have been chosen, each one with a definitive problem in aesthetic plastic surgery. The reasoning and solution I chose were considered both individually and so that this experience might contribute to method selection for more severe deformities.

Secondary Otoplasty

Although secondary rhinoplasty has received voluminous attention, little has been published about secondary ear repair, and it is still a relatively virgin field. Some principles have been published, but little detail.

Academically, secondary auriculoplasty includes both general and surgical trauma that needed correction to look lifelike and to be acceptable, as a result of our expertise. However, I would prefer to avoid semantics of classification, and focus on detailed diagnosis, detailed treatment, and adequate late control.

This young physician had been operated on twice when he was a boy to correct his prominent ears. Now the problem is not only the surgical sequelae but also the diagnosis.

The plan was to operate on one severely deformed ear at a time, starting with the left side. It was calculated to be long, tedious, and demanding surgery, requiring considerable sedation and local anesthesia. The result had to satisfy an already deeply frustrated patient, after two previous surgical disappointments. There could be no risking pressure ulceration or necrosis, due to surgery, bandaging, or position while asleep, during the postoperative period, in spite of dealing with already considerably scarred tissue. The whole situation was carefully discussed with the patient.

Childhood photographs show that his original deformity looked better when viewed from the front (Fig. 2), but adult side views (Fig. 3) and projection from the head (Figs. 4A and 4B) illustrate the gross defects.

To establish diagnosis, the defects had to be categorized to analyze every detail. First, it was obvious that the normal proportion of the three equal vertical segments (Fig. 5) as previously specified by this author,* did not exist. The middle third outdimensioned both the upper and lower thirds (upper, 13 mm; middle, 30 mm; lower, 11 mm). Second, it was an abnormally small ear, a mild microtia (Fig. 5), and expansion was needed.

---

*Davis JE. *Aesthetic and Reconstructive Otoplasty*. New York: Springer-Verlag; 1987.

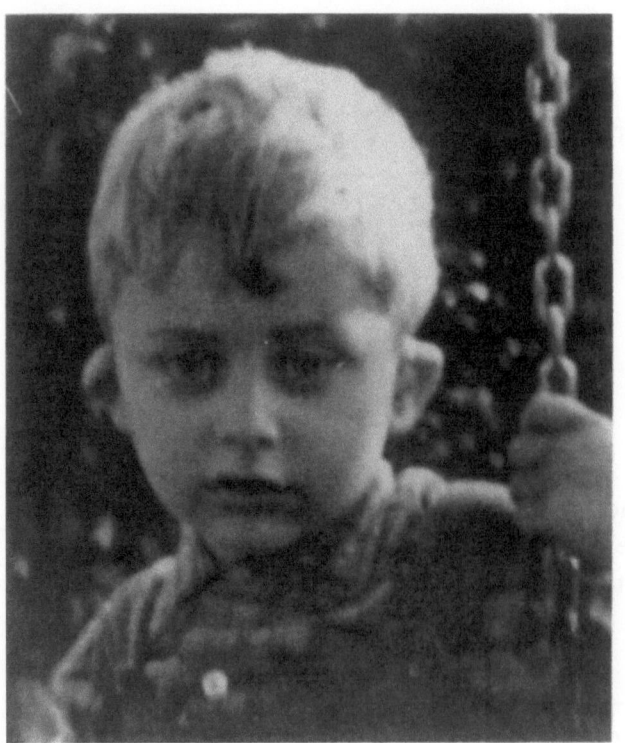 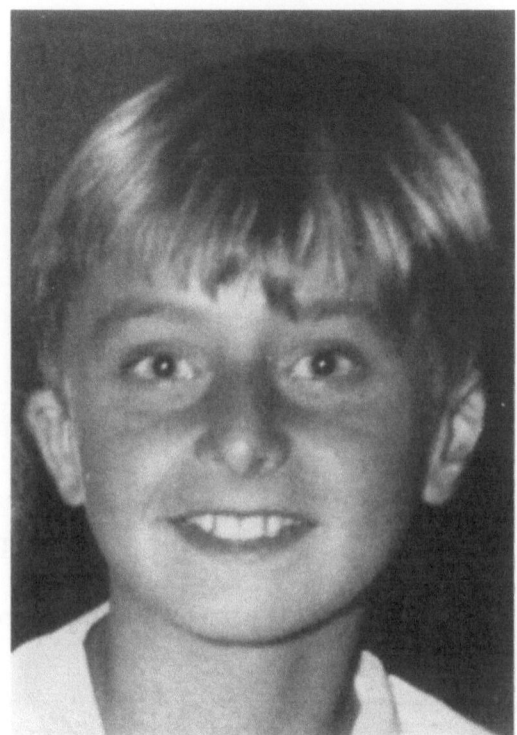

Figure 2

Where? How? The priority deformity was the overall shape of the upper third. It was essentially a "satyr" ear. The basic defect—insufficient scapha—remained and had become worse with forced flexion of the anthelix. The whole upper auricle gave the optical illusion of being tall and thin. It was not. It was short and thin. The scapha lacked height as well as width. The helix that circled around it was insufficient.

Third, the fossa triangularis was quite deformed (Fig. 5), especially due to the upward slant of the lower crus; also, the upper crus had a serrated overlap of the previously incised chondral edges.

Figure 3

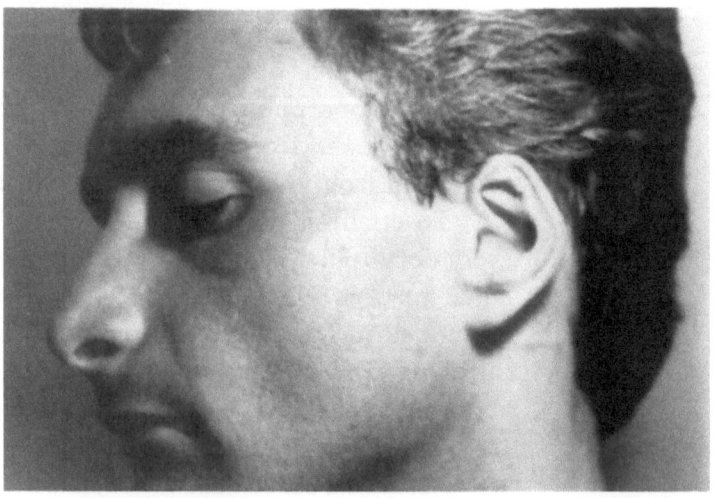

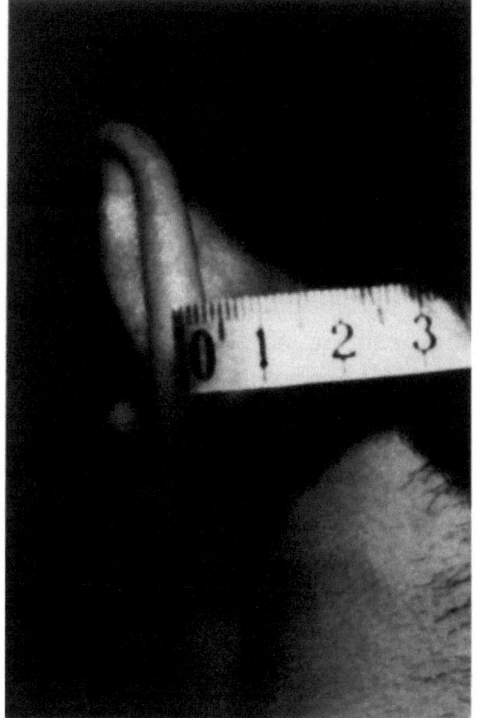
Figure 4A

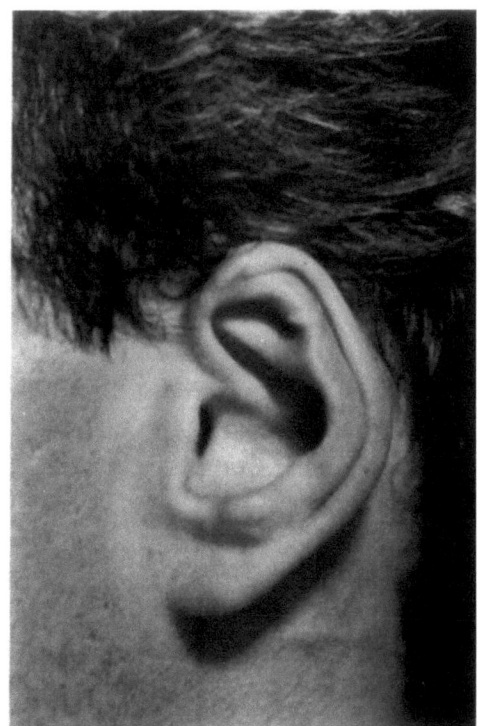
Figure 4B

Fourth, the whole posterior conchal wall remained very high, 20 mm helix-mastoid distance, and still caused ear prominence (Fig. 4A). The three factors together—high posterior conchal wall, lower crus slant, and ptotic antitragus—insufficiently surrounded the very large, wide open, gaping concha. The last two factors failed to curl in and partially close the concha.

Fifth, the antitragus was jutting out, prominent and ptotic, falling over a horizontally narrow and small lobule (Fig. 5).

Surgery commenced by incising along the previous posteromedial skin scar (Fig. 6). Care was taken to go straight down to the cartilaginous sur-

Figure 5

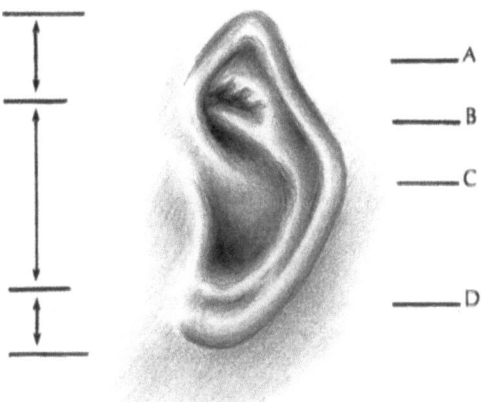

Secondary Otoplasty

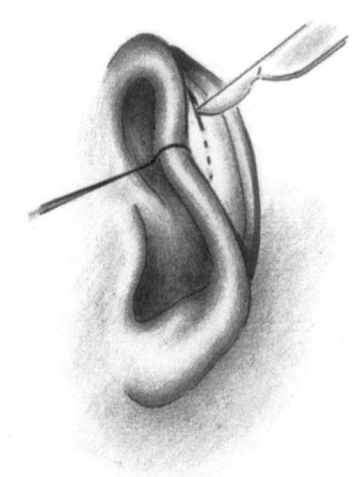

Figure 6

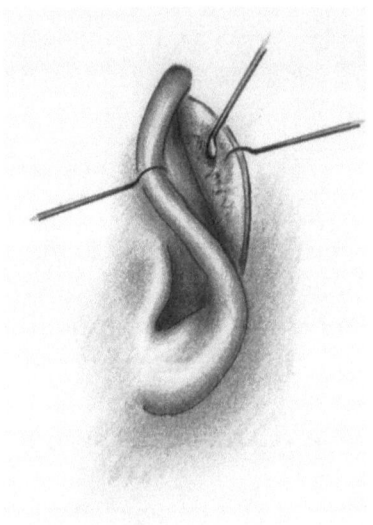

Figure 7

face, and then undermine over the perichondrium. There was considerable skin-to-cartilage adhesion due to abundant fibrous tissue in the subcutaneous fat, and gross cartilaginous irregularities. Once the cartilage was bared, guide transfixion dye points were pierced exactly along the helical sulcus base, needled through from the anterolateral surface. Only the cartilage was incised along these guide marks, with care taken to keep the anterolateral soft tissues intact.

The scaphal cartilage was retracted backward and the helix forward (Fig. 7). The anterolateral scaphal surface was carefully dissected, because it was found to be very irregular, having been cut, sliced, and overlapped in an attempt to forcibly bend the area until it was a mass of distorted fragments. The dissection was done with maximum precision, and the best instruments to do it were middle ear elevators, from sharp to semisharp, under magnification. The undermining was continued over the helix and lower crus, and both scaphal surfaces were bared. Both anterolateral and posteromedial soft tissues were very carefully preserved.

Needles with dye were used to transfix the guide points for conchal cartilage removal, to reduce the posterior conchal wall prominence (Fig. 8), as has been previously described by this author.* The conchal floor cartilage that was excised was kept to be used later as a graft.

Below the conchal cartilage, the local auricularis posterior muscle was also removed down to the mastoid fascia, to deepen the conchal floor while reducing the posterior wall prominence. By combining these two maneuvers for satisfactory relief, the convolutions harmonized. Conchal floor skin and subcutaneous tissue were kept intact and undivided, to spread over the new conchal bed.

By keeping the dissection to the perichondrium plane, there was minimal bleeding. However, pinpoint microcoagulation under magnification allowed a bloodless field to be obtained.

Figure 8

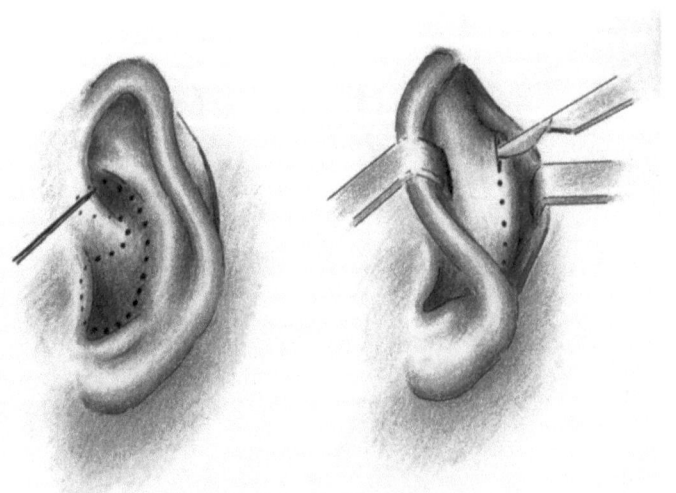

*Davis JE. *Aesthetic and Reconstructive Otoplasty.* New York; Heidelberg. Springer-Verlag, 1987.

Figure 9

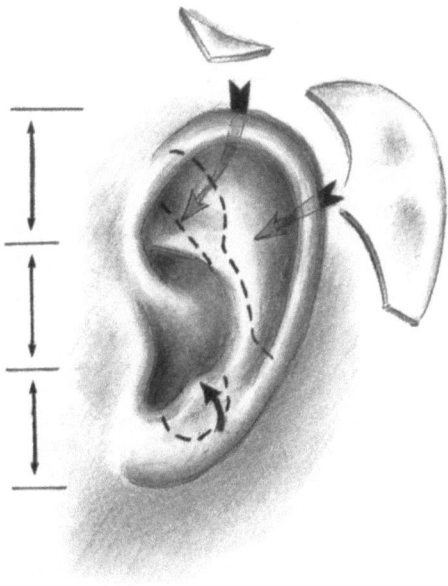

The conchal cartilage floor that had been removed was prepared to be used as a graft (Fig. 9). The severely deformed scaphal cartilage was discarded completely. The conchal cartilage graft was precisely shaped to fit into the defect after scaphal excision, but the height and width were increased to be in keeping with normal auricular dimensions. Remaining minor irregularities of parallel incisions along the anthelix that gave sharp borders were shaved down and pared to an even curvature. The cartilage graft was meticulously sutured into place, cartilage border to cartilage border, with 6-0 silk.

A surplus triangle of cartilage graft, with its curvature adjusted, was cut to bring down the slanted lower crus to a normal position, and shape the fossa triangularis. It was held in place in its skin socket with 6-0 silk transfixion sutures.

The prominent and everted antitragus was moved up and inward with the method previously described by this author.*

These cartilage corrections have been slightly exaggerated in Figure 9 to emphasize the concept of repair.

Then the skin flap was draped back over the new framework and the wound closed, with a minidrain placed for 72 hours. Antiseptic Vaseline wool was gently packed into the ear convolutions now shaped, and held with the very lightest dressing of elastic net.

The postoperative course was uneventful.

The result is shown in Figures 10 and 11. Compared with preoperative measurements, the major vertical axis had increased 6 mm (from 54 to 60 mm) and the width 12 mm (from 21 to 33 mm).

The conchal cavity had been reduced in size by bringing down the

---

*Davis JE. *Aesthetic and Reconstructive Otoplasty.* New York; Heidelberg. Springer-Verlag; 1987.

Figure 10

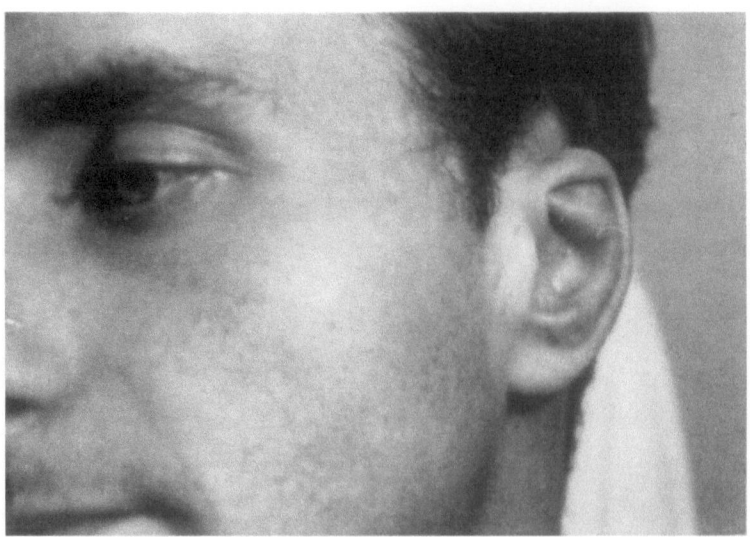

lower crus, incurling the antitragus, and reducing the prominence. The proportion of vertical segmental measurements had radically improved (upper, 19 mm; middle, 20 mm; lower, 19 mm) so that they were practically equal and in keeping with calculated harmony.

The expansion was quite evident. Ear convolutions had been shaped, normal curvatures had appeared, with closer to ideal overall aesthetics. The ear-to-head relationship was satisfactory, as the helix-mastoid prominence had been reduced from 20 to 14 mm.

The change is evident in the pre- and postoperative photographs. Figure 12 shows the result at 4 years. One detail is especially worth men-

Figure 11

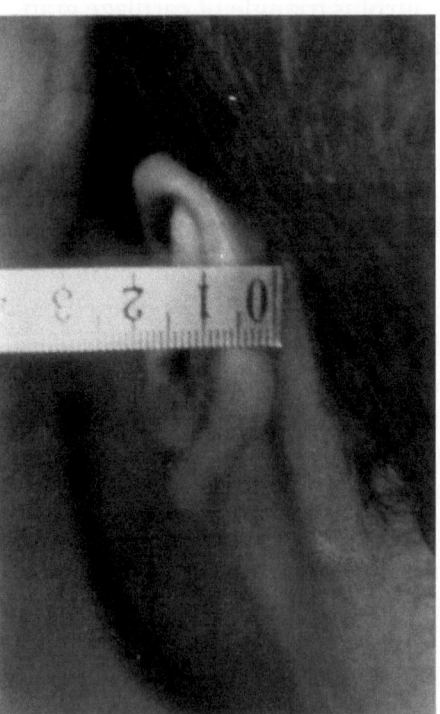 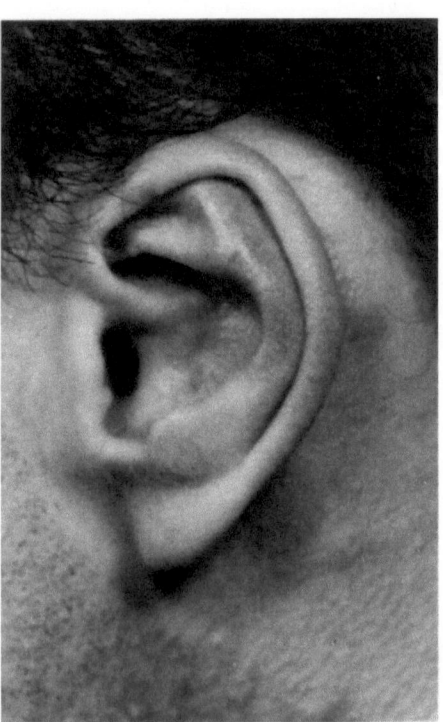

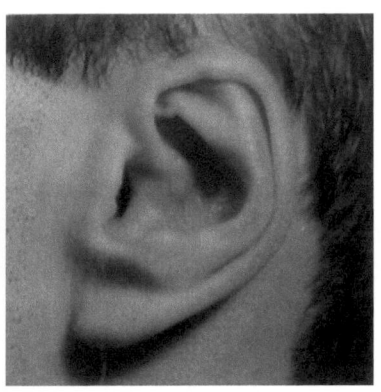

Figure 12

tioning: Observe that the lobule was retroplaced when compared with the preoperative condition. The reason was that with the expanded scapha, the encircling helix was short. When draped over the dome it became very tight and dragged the upper ear down with its tautness, and it deformed the area. Thus, the upper helix had to be thoroughly relaxed. The anterior helix could not be used, because the radix held up the dome and the lower crus and fossa triangularis in position. So the helical "give" had to come from the cauda helicis and the lobular laxity, after the fashion of Antia.* This is an example of auricular "halo" performing as a unit, by rotating around the "core."† The laxity was taken from lobe to dome.

The second side was shaped and progressed similarly.

Conchal Flap

Modifications of the conchal floor composite flap‡ have been found useful. The following example illustrates the use of the remaining upper third to crest the dome. The result of this patient's mild dog bite was a severe infection (Fig. 13). The result of the chondritis was loss of the upper auricular third. The patient came in for a simple repair. He got it (Figs. 14 to 17): the result of one operation (Fig. 16). My offer to reposition the radix helicis was complacently refused.

Surprising!

Figure 13

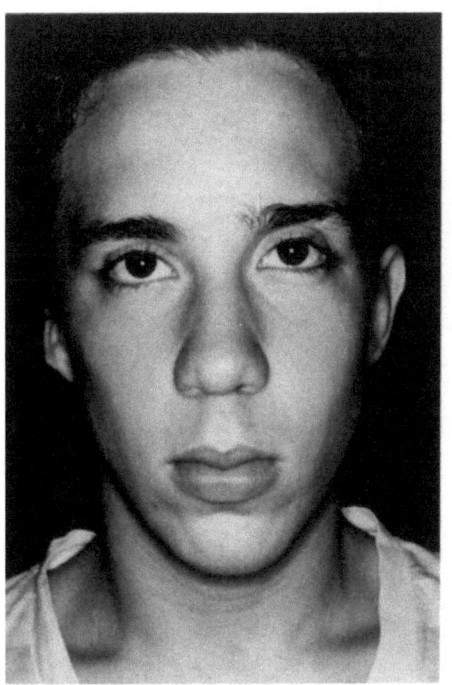
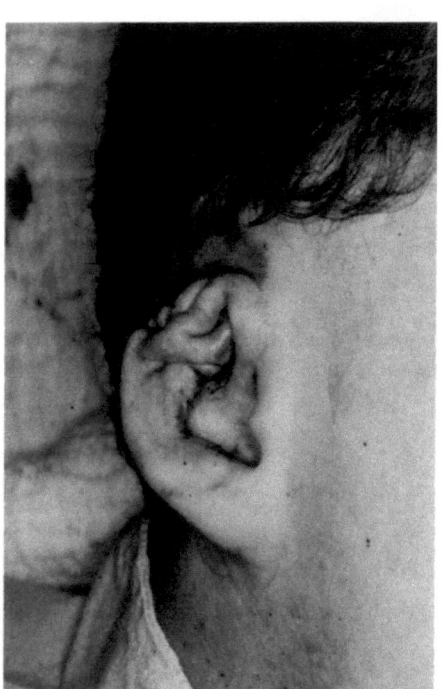

---

*From Antia N.H. and Buch V.I. Plast. Reconstr. Surg. 39:472, 1967.

†Davis JE. *Aesthetic and Reconstructive Otoplasty.* New York; Springer-Verlag, 1987.

‡Davis JE. *Aesthetic and Reconstructive Otoplasty.* New York; Heidelberg. Springer-Verlag; 1987.

Cryptotia and Satyr Ear

In my experience cryptotia has been frequently associated with satyr ear (Fig. 17). The following case is an example (Fig. 18). This 8-year-old boy was bilaterally affected, especially evident when seen from the back.

The shape of the ears was studied by relaxing the area, and then manually bringing out the auricle from under the scalp, so that the upper pole was separated from the head. With the upper ear entirely on view, the aural details were registered. The satyr scaphoid fossa deficiency and helical drape were evident, with the mid-dome helical kink. However, when the patient became excited or expressive, the ears popped back under the scalp again. Synchronic action of both frontalis and auricularis superioris muscles has been reported by this author,* and attention has also been brought to the auricularis superioris in cryptotia by Torikai et al.†

The Davis test was performed by raising the eyebrows forcefully; the auricularis superioris muscles were contracted simultaneously with the frontalis, and the auricularis dragged the upper auricular pole inward under the scalp.

On further examining the auricularis muscles, it was found that they were inserted higher than normal, into the scapha apart from the concha, and the muscular contraction dragged the auricular cartilage in and under the cephalic scalp skin.

The degree of re-dislocation and the effect of this muscular contraction was carefully gauged for later surgical SMAS correction. Thus, the sur-

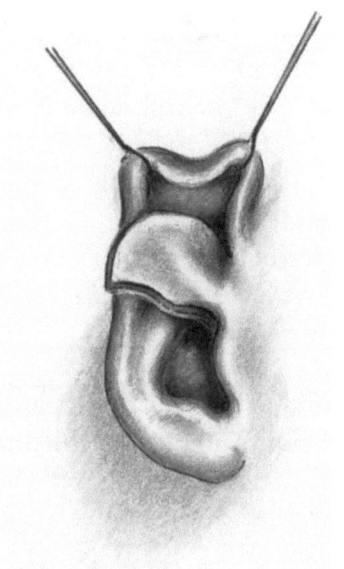

Figure 14

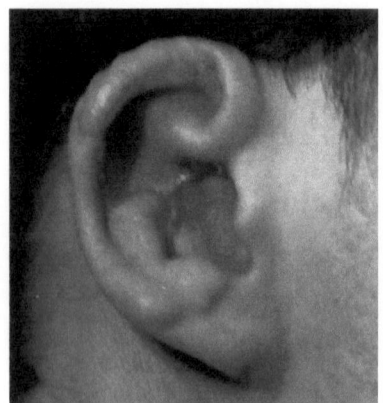

Figure 16

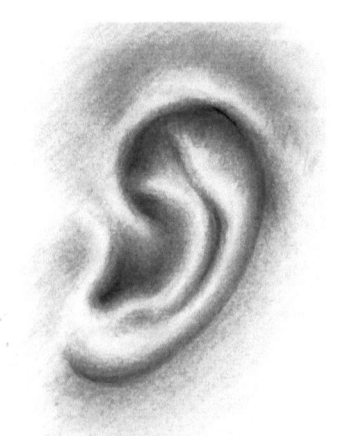

Figure 17

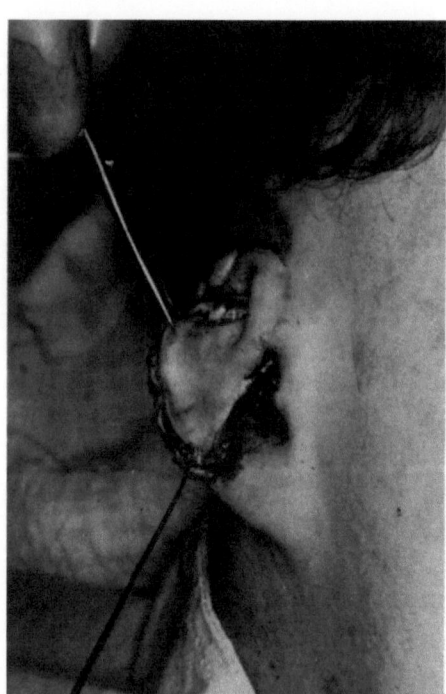
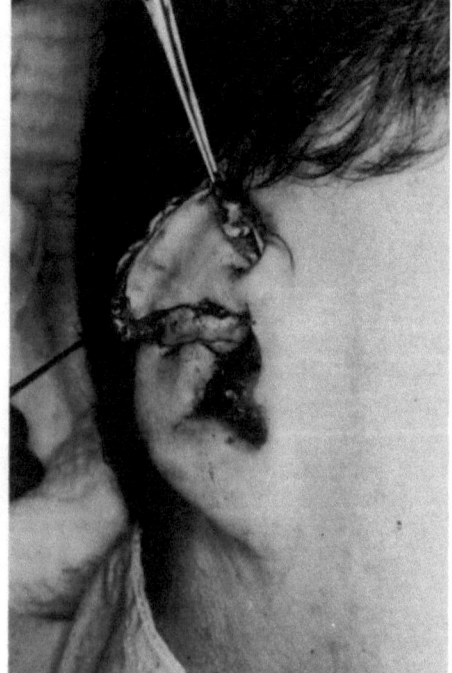

Figure 15

---

*Davis JE. *Aesthetic and Reconstructive Otoplasty.* New York; Springer-Verlag; 1987.

†Torikai K, Ando S, Yoshida T, Asano T, Matsumoto Y, Anze M. Anatomy of the auricular muscles and its surgical application. *Jpn J Plast Reconstruct Surg.* 1982;25:46.

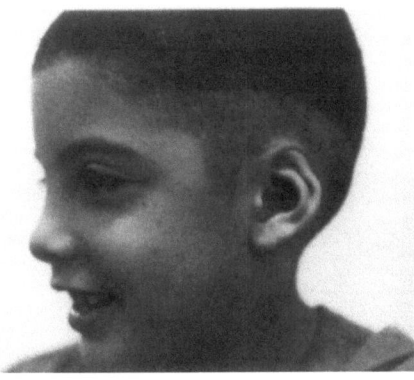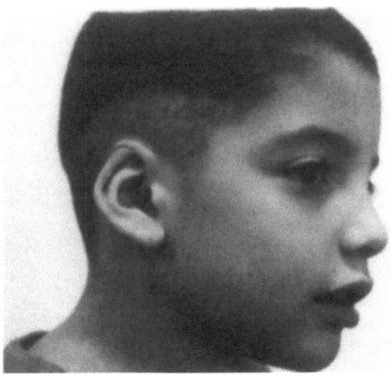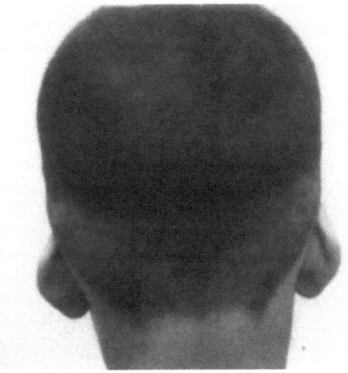

Figure 18

geon could calculate the necessary type of myotomy or myomectomy of the auricularis superioris.

Understanding the mechanism of cryptotia is important. The auricularis superioris muscle has been found inserted high into the scaphal cartilage, and its contraction drew the chondral dome up and inward toward the skull, and then under the scalp. This dislocation recurred with each frontalis muscular contraction, but the auricle slipped out again into its normal position when the muscle was relaxed and the patient combed the ear out from under the scalp.

Repetition of this slipping back and forth mechanism created gliding and lax fascia tissue formation around the cartilage, which further aided the deformity. The upper auricle was gradually drawn in toward the head as a dominant position and shape, which was evident when viewed from the front or back.

The satyr ingredient was frequent, including the upper helical overhang and the kink, due to overlapping embryonic hillocks 3 and 4 as a crease of triple cartilage layers, but the theoretical helical dome curve was preserved.

It was obvious that the scarcity of skin due to the cryptotia coincided with excess skin from the satyr drape. Surgery was planned to have one factor compensate for the other, so that a good overall shape could be obtained without invagination recurrence. The repair included correction both of auricular relief and permanent projection from the head, without residual foreign bodies.

Surgery commenced with the skin incision delineating a hairless superior flap, as illustrated (Fig. 19). The incision continued backward along the deepest depression of the auriculocephalic sulcus, which was very shallow.

The flap was brought away from the head, and the auricular border of the retroaural incision dissected over the perichondrium (Fig. 20). Dissection was continued over the helical dome; the cartilage dome was laid bare on the outer surface, but both lateral and medial surfaces of the drape were denuded. Soft superficial tissues were very carefully kept intact and in continuity with the previous triangular flap.

Then the excess cartilaginous overhang was removed and the kink shaved down until it pared along with the rest of the helical dome (Fig. 21).

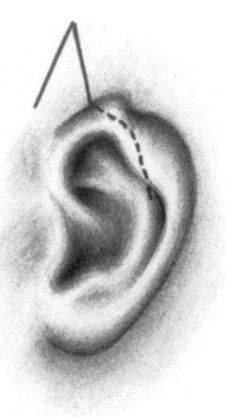 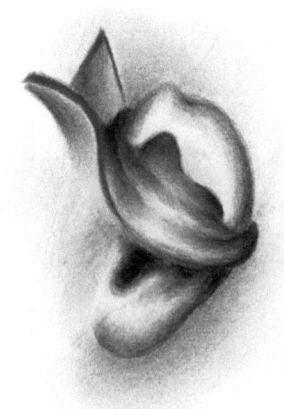 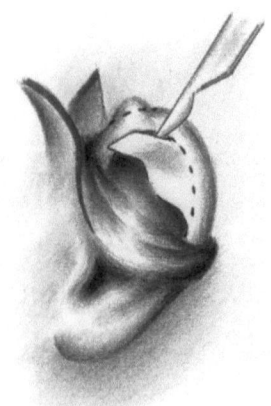

Figure 19 **Figure 20** **Figure 21**

Thus, the helical border became even, regular, and in continuity with the rest of the helix.

When the cartilage was retracted and brought away from the head, the tensed auricularis superioris muscle came into view (Fig. 22). It was observed that the subcutaneous fat had formed a pocket of lax tissue similar to a hernia formation. The scissors passed under the muscle, and it was resected. Also the gliding tissue was removed. The causes of cryptotia were thus removed, and the upper auricular cartilage was no longer held anchored to the cephalic surface by the muscle band. The upper auricular pole then stood normally away from the head.

It was important also to deepen the postaural sulcus, beyond the conchal limit. Two different flaps were used. The previous triangular flap was brought back to cover the cephalic surface and sutured into place (Fig. 23).

But the overhang skin was gently stretched and draped back over the helical dome and posteromedial auricular aspect, advancing deep down into the sulcus. The skin was sufficiently abundant that on rotating and advancing (Fig. 23) it formed a small dog-ear at the upper angle that was snipped off and sutured. No skin graft was necessary.

Figure 22 **Figure 23**

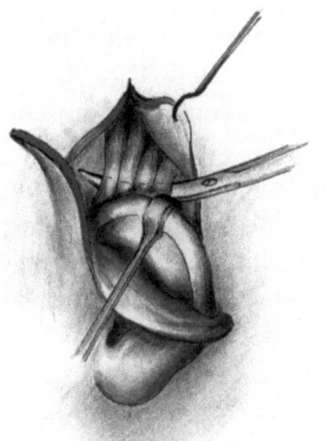 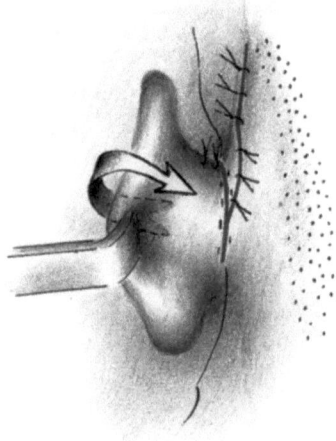

Figure 24

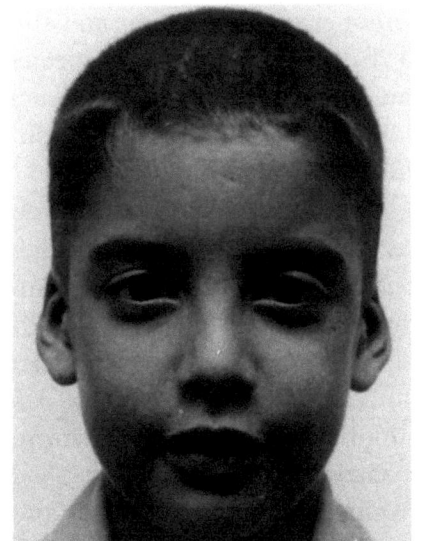
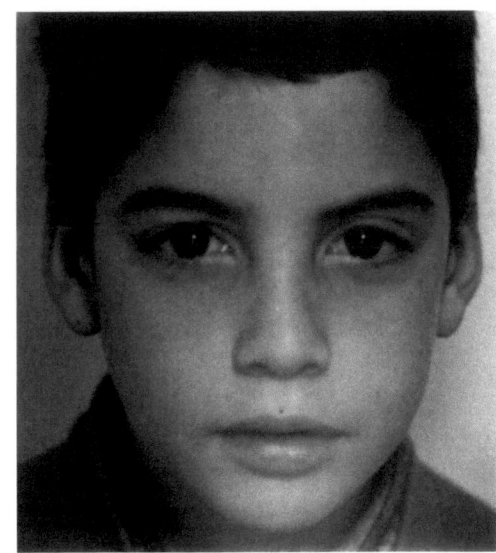

Figure 25

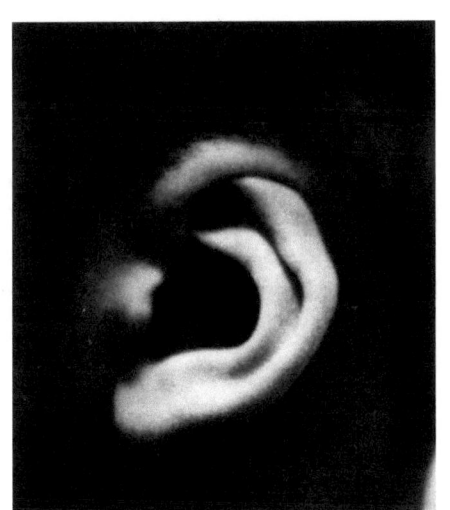
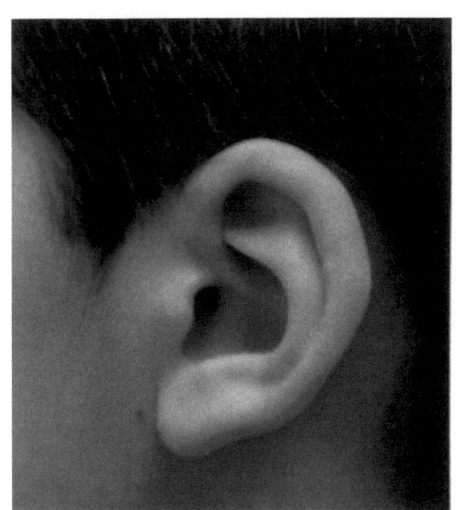

Figure 26

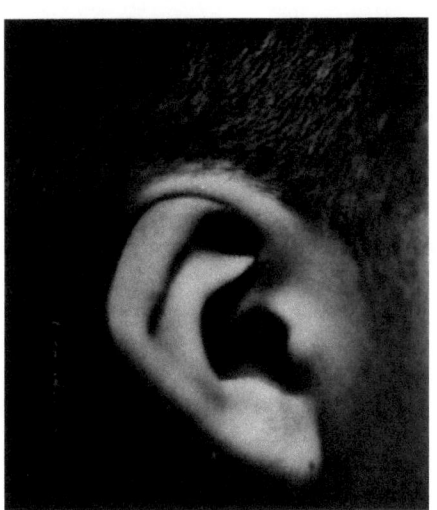
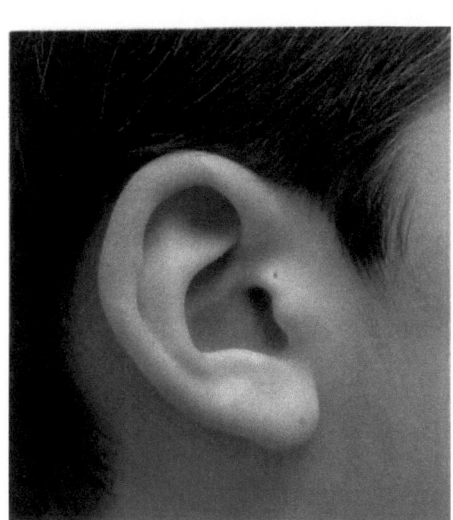

The preoperative condition and the postoperative results are shown (Figs. 24 to 26). Adequate upper ear projection from the head was obtained. The retroaural sulcus remained deep along its entire length, and the invagination did not recur. Improvement in shape is shown and has remained unaltered for 5 years.

Trauma

Conchal cartilage is the ideal skeletal support for traumatic ear loss, especially the upper auricle (Fig. 27). The following case was repaired in two operations. The contralateral conchal cartilage was lodged in the first stage (Fig. 28), and at the second stage the ear was raised with a retroaural skin graft and midhelical correction performed. Full size, flexibility, and elasticity were obtained (Fig. 29).

This young woman had been in an automobile crash one month before. A crossed bite and condylar neck fracture had been diagnosed, and she was being prepared for maxillofacial surgery. Her ear on the same side had been ripped off, and she had a subtotal avulsion of the auricle. I suggested that she commence with ear repair, and await the spontaneous fracture outcome, considering the posttraumatic period that had elapsed, before embarking on temporomandibular joint surgery (Fig. 30).

She was an air hostess, and these jobs are in demand. Competition is fierce. She was denied permission to fly without an ear. This weighed the scales, and auriculoplasty priority was decided.

The auricular wound had healed. The exact piece of missing ear was illustrated as a "ghost," and used for precision surgical planning (Fig. 31).

The remaining and partly amputated concha was not used as material for repair, but kept entirely as the foundation for both framework and lobular reconstruction.

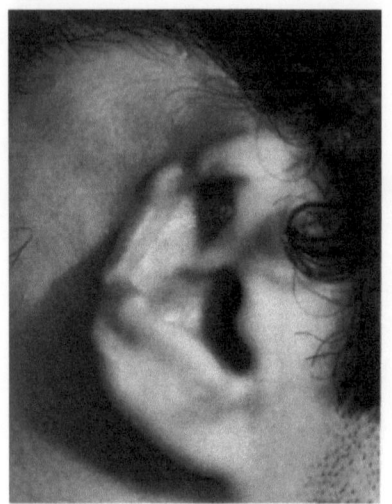

Figure 27

Figure 28

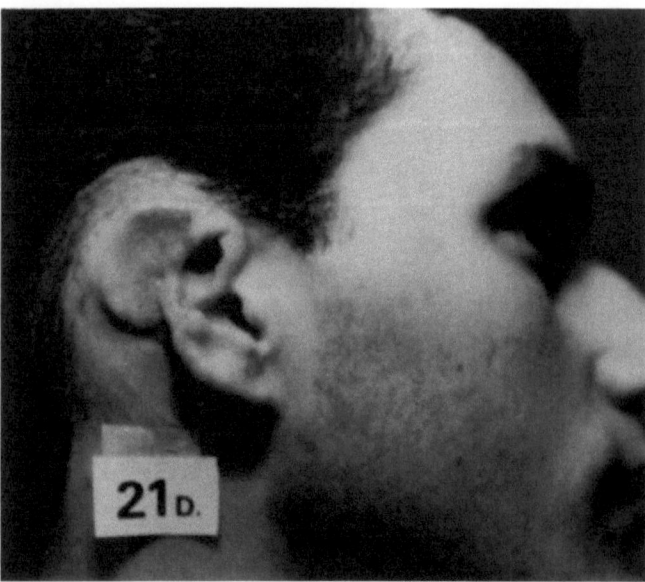
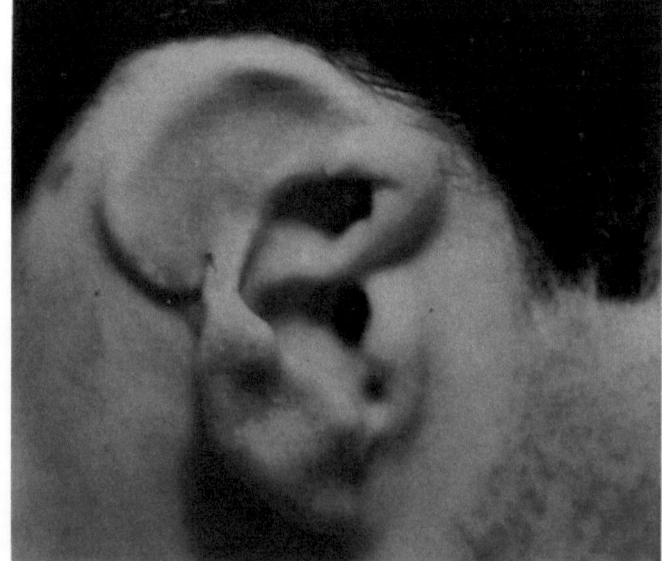

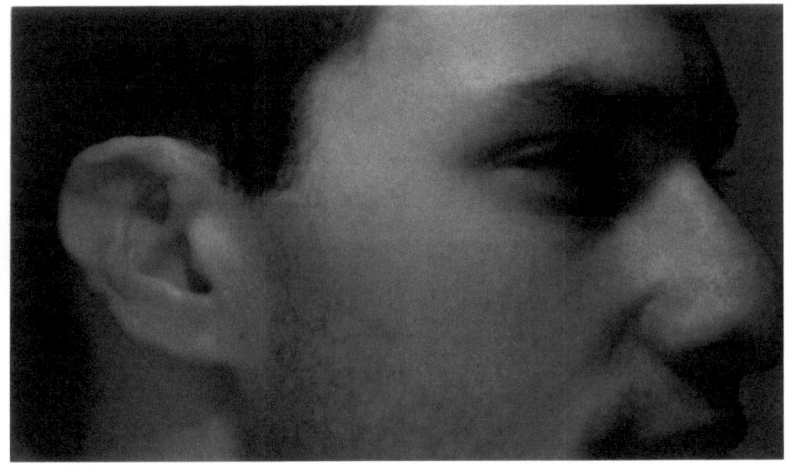
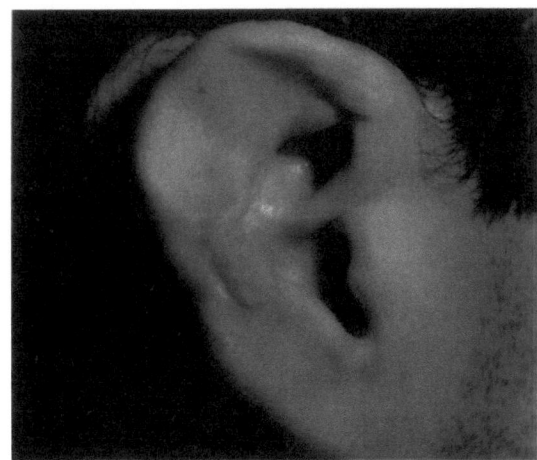

Figure 29

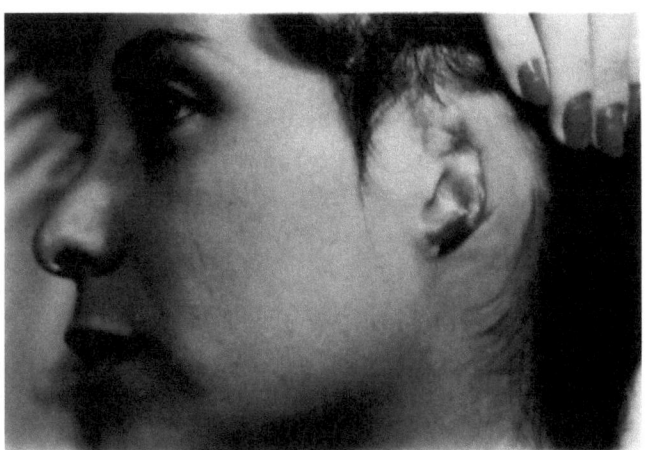
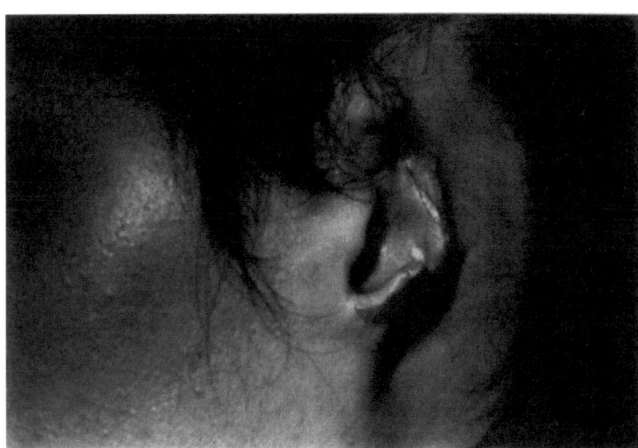

Figure 30

Figure 31

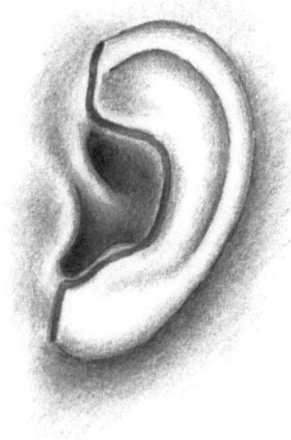

Reconstruction commenced with revision of the scar, and grafting in conchal cartilage from the normal side, through a border hairline approach (Fig. 32). The conchal cartilage was carefully tailored, with two segments sutured together, to fill the defect precisely. It was inserted immediately under a skin thickness flap to obtain the maximum delicacy and relief definition. The cartilage graft border was held firmly in contact with the amputated conchal cartilage border by transfixion sutures through the concha and tied over a bolus, to keep the framework in place.

Forty days later the second stage was performed. The conchal cartilage had grafted well, and the cartilage-to-cartilage apposition was held (Fig. 33). The scapha and helix were to be raised, and simultaneously the lobule was to be reconstructed.

The upper framework was raised, and excess skin flap wrapped around the helical border (Fig. 34). The flap extended anteriorly and down, and was enough to supplement the anterior helix, and the roll was held in place with a Z-plasty arrowheaded into the radix helicis (Fig. 35).

The lower ear was formed by three flaps, each independent in size, shape, thickness, movement of displacement, and blood supply. The ante-

Figure 32

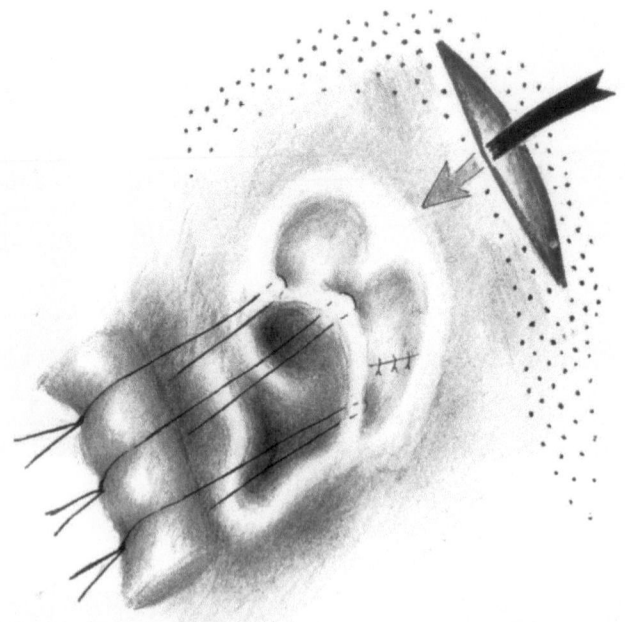

rior flap was shaped as a large normally positioned lobule, kept fat, and undermined to the lower antitragal cartilage border. The posterior flap was turned forward and swung around and under the lobular flap, to line it. The relatively narrow pedicle allowed it to roll easily into place, and it was held with gentle transfixion sutures surfaced at the antitragal gutter.

The third and lower flap was a rhytidectomy advancement. Dissection was carried quite extensively down the neck, keeping the flap thin enough to enhance good advancement, allowing it then to be brought right up behind the neoauricle to the hairline, without tension, over the mastoid. Skin

Figure 33

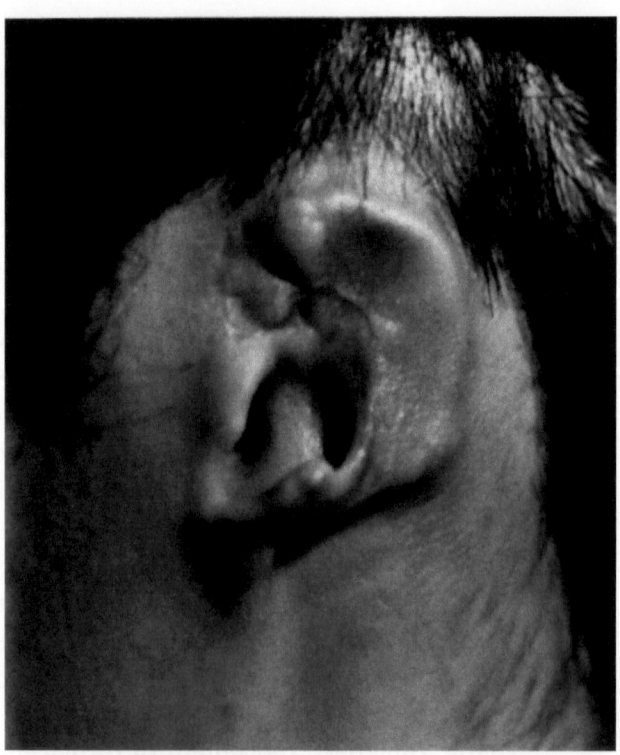

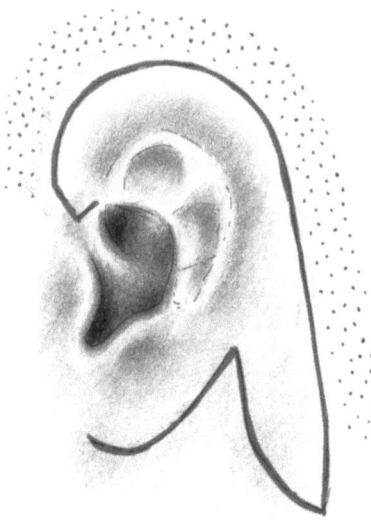

Figure 34

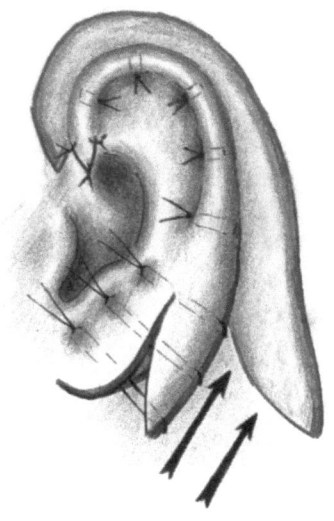

Figure 35

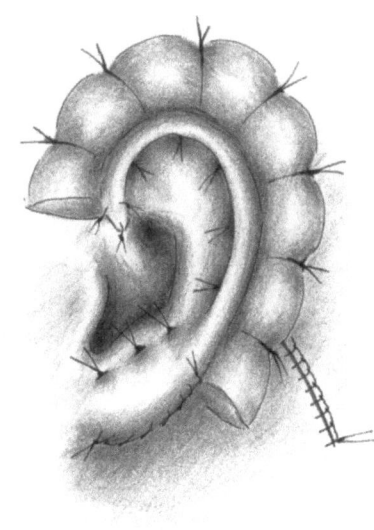

Figure 36

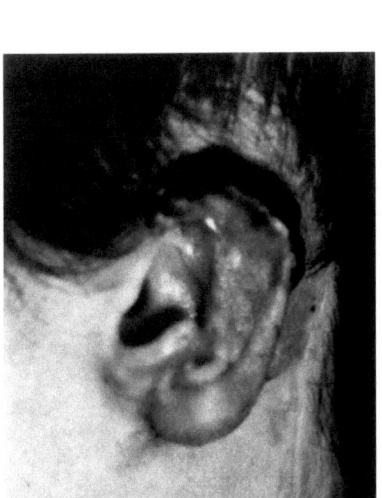

Figure 37

Figure 38

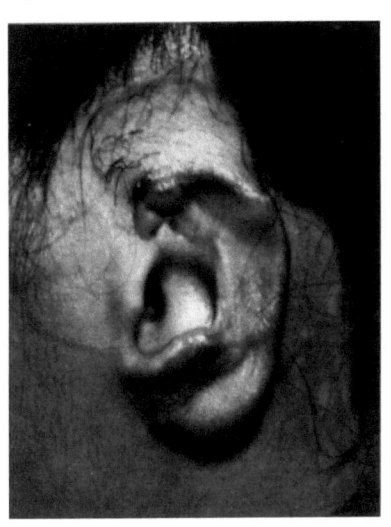

grafts were avoided in this area, so that the normal texture remained visible.

The residual upper raw surface was covered with an inguinal skin graft of intermediate thickness, held in place with a tie-on Böhler bolus dressing (Fig. 36).

The two first flaps were carefully sutured together at the free border of the neolobule with 7-0 silk, after cautious vascular control (Fig. 36).

The postoperative progress of the lobule and rhytidectomy was excellent, but the helical dome became cyanotic and 2-mm border necrosis took place (Fig. 37). As previous experience with this method had been good, and during surgery the circulation had been perfect, this outcome was surprising.

Then I discovered that the patient had been secretly chain smoking during the postoperative period. Much has been written in general surgery, and some in plastic surgery, about the circulatory dangers in smokers, but nothing in auricular reconstruction. So beware!

Hyperbaric oxygenation was very useful.

Second intention healing left no cartilage loss, but the irregularly scarred skin created an ugly helical dome (Fig. 38). The result at this stage, however, was sufficient for her to be permitted to resume working as a hostess.

But the helical crest was irregular and needed added material. A mastoid bridge flap was taken from the previous retroaural skin graft, and slung across to cover the helix (Fig. 39) after the principle of Johann Dieffenbach, modified by Blair Rogers, and later published by John Converse* as the "tunnel" method.

The somewhat retroplaced lobule and high sharp antitragus needed improvement, so this was associated with the helical dome revision. The lob-

---

*Converse JM. Acquired deformities of the auricle. Tunnel procedure. In: *Reconstructive Plastic Surgery*. Philadelphia: W.B. Saunders; 1964:1114.

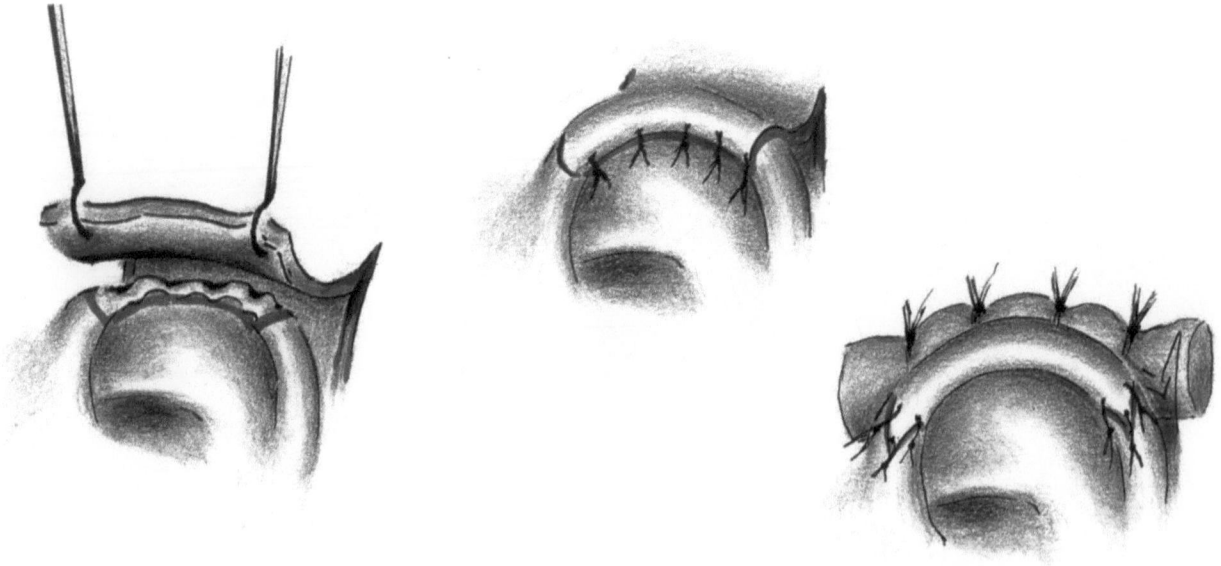

Figure 39

ule was shifted forward with the method described by this author,* and the deformed antitragus trimmed at the same time (Fig. 40).

As the patient stopped smoking, the progress was uneventful. The pedicle was severed, maintaining a bulky upper helix, and the helical ends were Z-plastied to avoid circular scar contractures. The cephalic donor site was again skin grafted.

Figure 40

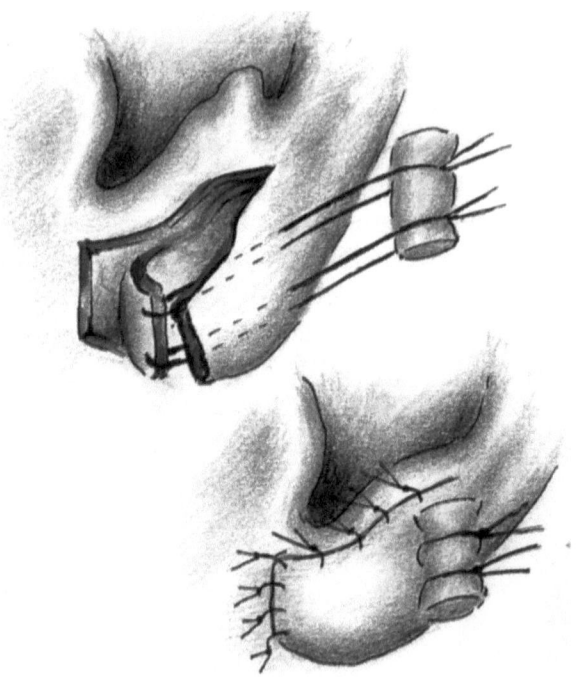

*Davis JE. *Aesthetic and Reconstructive Otoplasty*. New York; Springer-Verlag; 1987.

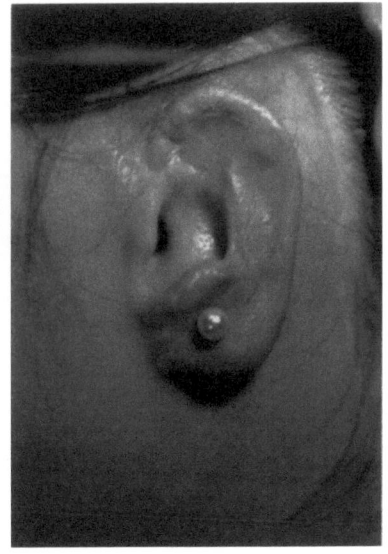

Figure 41

In 6 months the bulky dome had subsided, and the helical border had normalized.

Later, the lobe was perforated with an earring (Fig. 41).

The temporomandibular joint spontaneously progressed well, allowing the patient to rotate and open her mouth without pain or limitation of motion.

The earring she is wearing demonstrates the depth of the sublobular sulcus (Fig. 42). Auricular size is sufficient (Fig. 42). Flexibility and elasticity are shown. Transillumination marks the degree of delicacy (Fig. 43).

Recovery of nerve supply has been undescribed so far in auriculoplasty. Good trophic texture, circulatory response, sweating, and other protopathic sensation appeared after 6 months. But double pinpoint discrimination (6 mm) and cotton wool touch for epicritic sensation were not normal and symmetrical with the other side until 20 months after repair (Fig. 44). Full sensation (subsidiary, tickle, erogenous, reflex) were complete in 24 months.

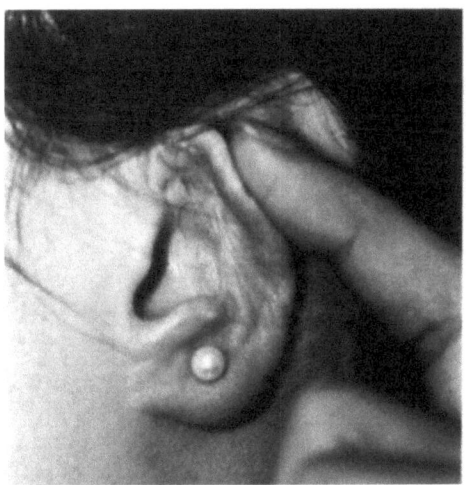
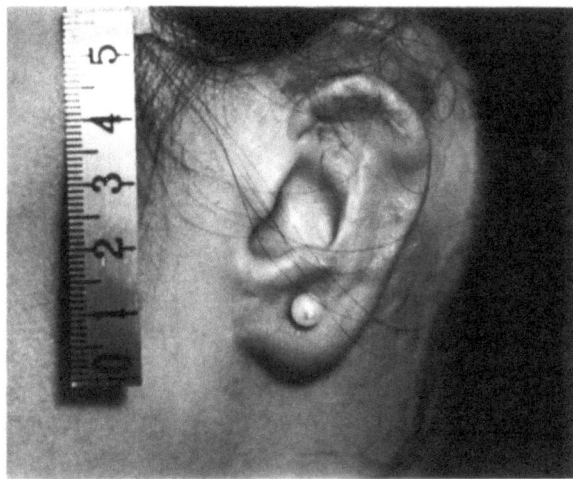

Figure 42

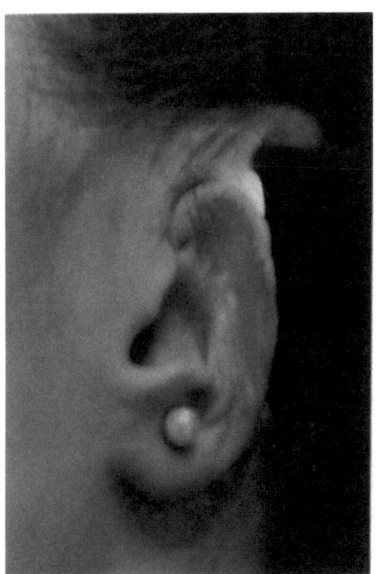

Figure 43

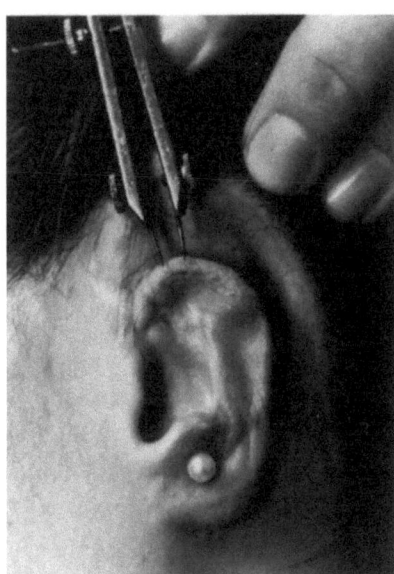
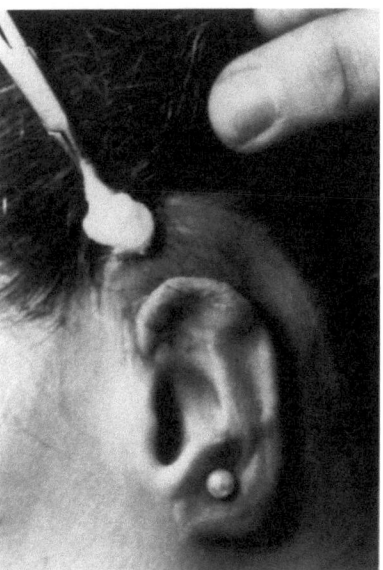

Figure 44

Trauma

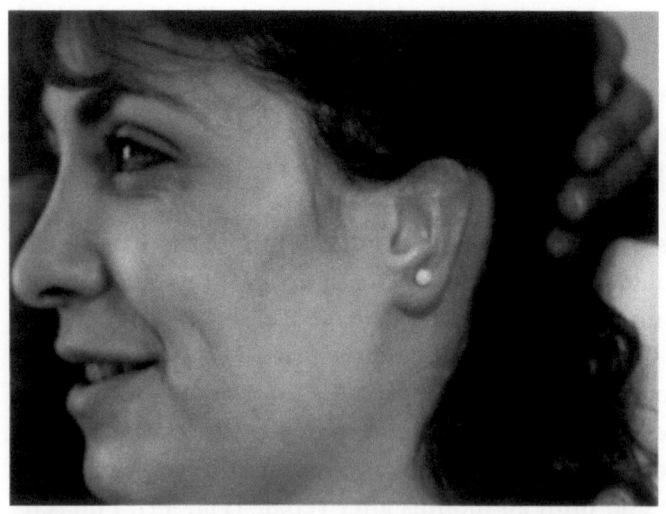 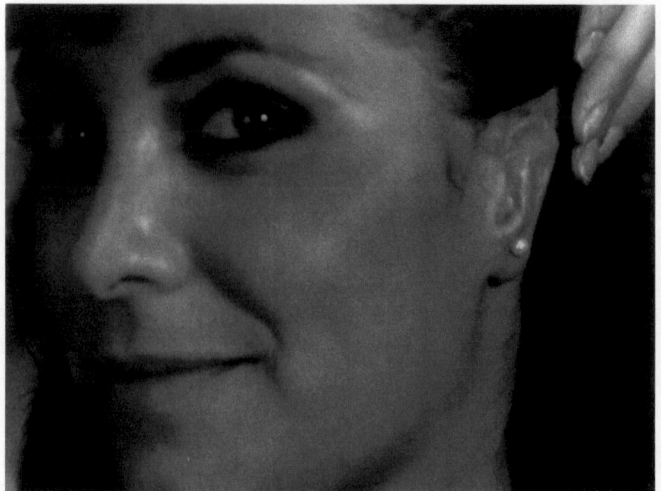

Figure 45

The big happy smile she has in (Fig. 45) is the result. In fact, she was getting married the next day. I had asked her partner, who had driven the car during the accident, if he felt indebted, if he had guilt feelings. He emphatically answered "No!" and reminded me that he was a pilot and that risk factors were a part of his work. True love is a rare treasure.

She now wears high hair styles.

Healing Potential

Reconstruction involves two stages: the actual surgery and the healing process. Both are equally important. The first is directly under our control, but the second is not always so. Careful contributing treatment must be weighed. The following is such a case.

Keloids

Keloids are complex. This flame-burned patient had been rejected in several dermatologic and plastic surgery centers, because no one would guarantee results. He had burned his arm, hand, and face 4 years previously, but only the ear developed a keloid (Fig. 46). It had grown during the last year, was purple-red, with dilated capillaries, and was angry and itchy. Treatment with local corticoids and laser rays had been useless, and therefore surgery had not been considered.

The various factors in the makeup of this posttraumatic keloid pathology were explained to the patient, that the quality and technique of strontium beta therapy was as important as the surgery, and that complementary medical treatment should be administered.

Surgery was performed in the following way. With the patient under deep sedation and local anesthesia, the keloid was excised completely, as illustrated in Figure 47, until reaching normal skin and subcutaneous fat. It was observed that the keloid involved not only the postauricular skin that wrapped around the helix, but also a substantial layer of fibrous fatty tissue under the skin.

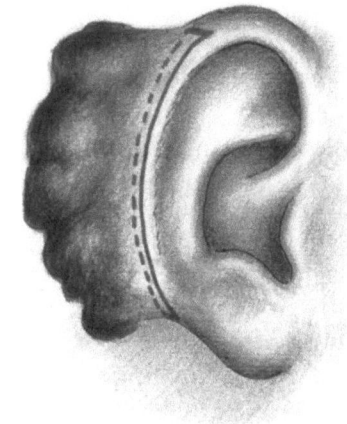 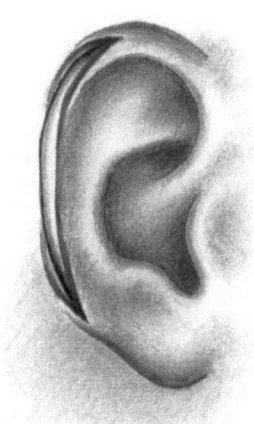 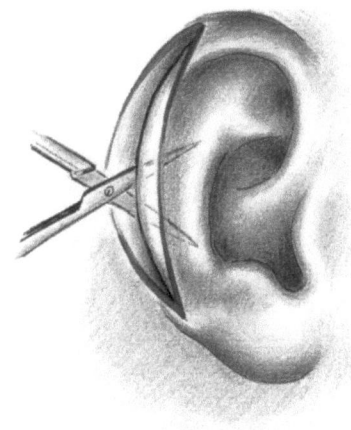

Figure 46 **Figure 47** **Figure 48**

The helical cartilage remained visible as the skin borders retracted. The first important point in this surgery is to avoid any tension of the suture line, and immediate direct suturing should not be done until adequate relaxation had been obtained. Suture tension is a dangerous factor in stimulating keloid recurrence.

Only the posterior wound border was undermined, and the plane of dissection was over the perichondrium. It was an easy plane and practically bloodless. Blunt dissection with fine scissors extended beyond the whole length of the wound (Fig. 48).

The undermining continued until reaching the auriculocephalic sulcus (Fig. 49), and then the posteromedial flap advanced well. It swept around the free helical cartilage border, until it fell spontaneously and gently into contact with the anterior wound edge (Fig. 50).

Before suturing, very careful pinpoint hemostasis was performed.

In contrast to the usual drainage site along the auriculocephalic sulcus, and because of the danger of keloidal formation in this area, a small

Figure 49 **Figure 50**

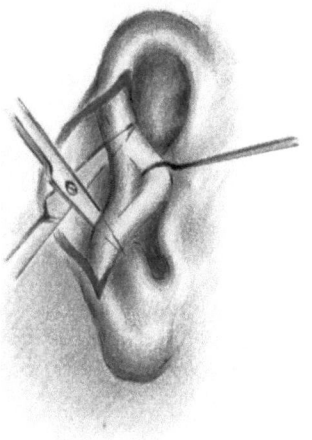 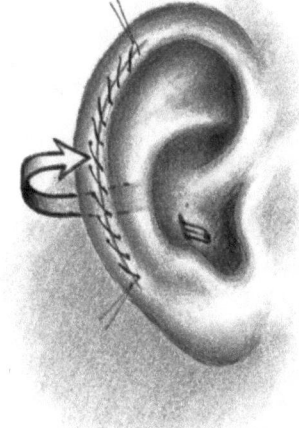

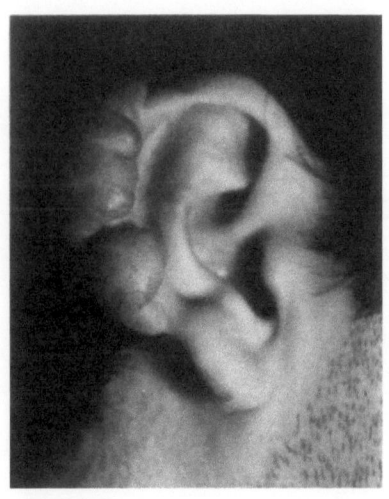

Figure 51

incision was stabbed through the antelateral conchal skin and cartilage to lodge a minimal drain in the wound cavity (Fig. 50). Thus, effusion collection under the flap was avoided, which ensured the cavity remaining adequately collapsed during the next 4 days. Then the drain was removed.

It is well to remember that conchal skin is skin in transition, halfway between mucosa and surface skin, and normal healing will take place without a keloid.

The helical skin wound was sutured, carefully appositioned with 7-0 silk, without tension and slack borders.

Beta therapy with strontium 90 was applied preoperatively with 333 cGy (four fields) 17, 12, and 8 days before surgery, totaling 999 cGy. Postoperatively 333 cGy (two fields) was administered 1, 3, 6, 9, 12, and 15 days after surgery, totaling 1998 cGy. A perikeloidal margin of 8 mm was the application limit. Very careful shielding of the unaffected tissue and the uniformity of ray treatment (we believe fractionation gives the best results) contribute to a successful result.

Severe neuroendocrinologic control supplied the complementary cushion. Neuroendocrine medication consisted of treatment of tertiary shock, which was considered to be a delayed suprarenal imbalance. Suprarenal stimulation was achieved indirectly by hypophyseal action via thyroid and gonadotrophic microdoses during 3 months postoperatively.

The final scar along the helical border was practically invisible, felt normal, and was not painful or itchy. Observe that no keloid appeared in the concha drainage site (without strontium therapy) and the scar was imperceptible (Fig. 54).

This is a spectacular example of helical skin behaving as postaural with marked keloid, while the concha had normal healing (Figs. 51 and 54).

Figure 52

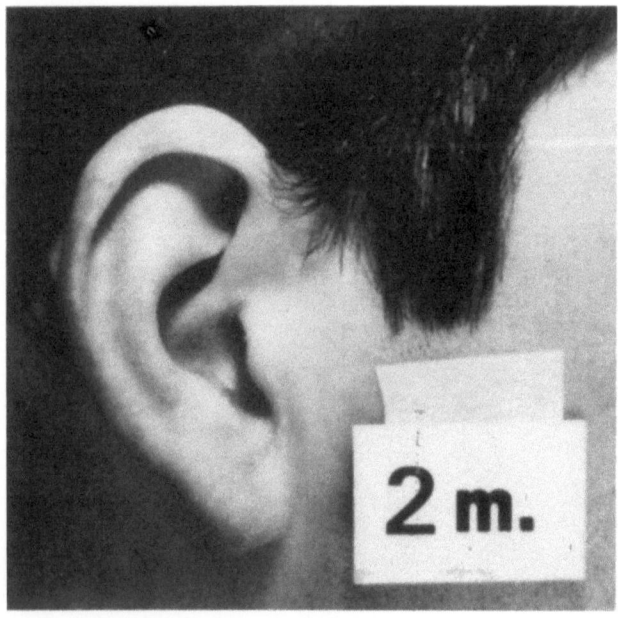
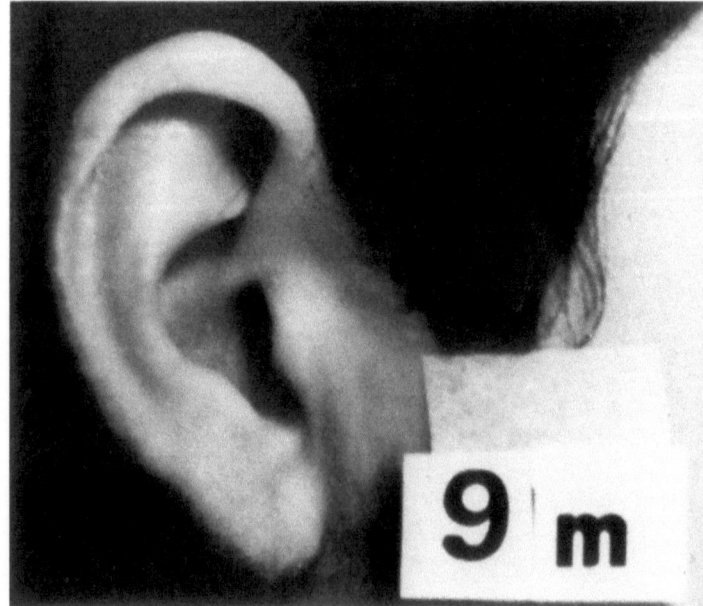

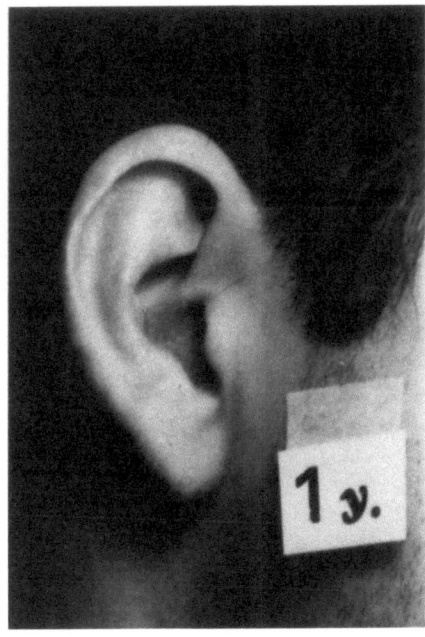
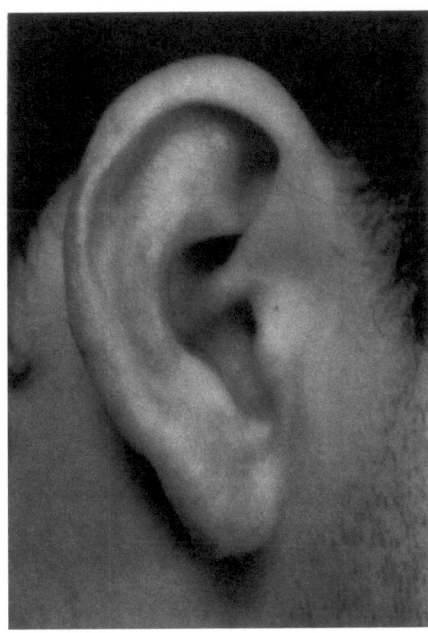
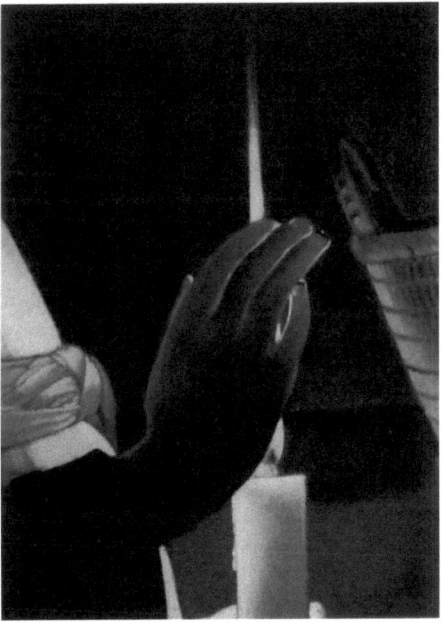

Figure 53

Figure 54
Final result

Figure 55

Test for Measurement of Delicacy

An ear is called nice, or pretty, or elegant because of its harmony. But it is attractive because of its delicacy. If delicacy is a necessary condition of the final result, how is it to be scientifically measured?

I have sought a way to measure and document auricular tissue texture delicacy. The following test has shown practical results.

A fragment of George de la Tour's (1593–1652) painting *Education of the Virgin*, from the Frick Collection, is shown in Figure 55 and is applied as a guide for transillumination, and the translucidity is photographed. It is interesting how much the surgeon can learn about details of his reconstruction by using this test, especially about the frame uniformity and soft tissue evenness. Its use in controlling the progress of postoperative de-swelling has been quite remarkable. Application of this test shows how transillumination can measure the delicacy of the final result (Fig. 56).

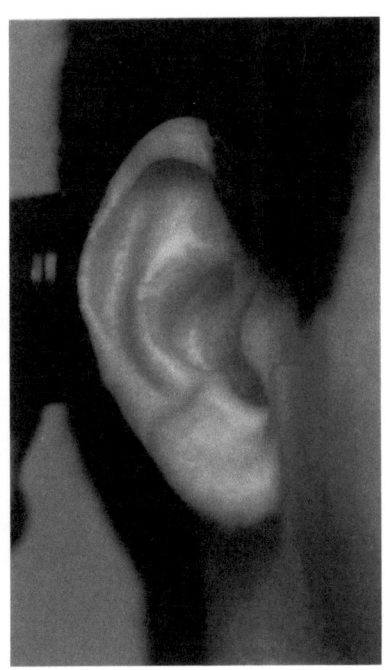

Figure 56

3
Moderate Microtia and Partial Atresia

Embryology of the External Ear

Clinical observations of collected deformities have led me to understand that present embryologic conceptions had to be thoroughly revised. So research was done by Gustavo Grgicevic, in the Chair of Human Anatomy, Buenos Aires University, and the Chair of Human Anatomy, Argentine Northeastern University.* Part of his findings have allowed him to "sectorize" the external ear, establishing anatomic and functional units of tissue constitution, growth, and pathology, while further observations have shed light on controversial issues that will be considered later.

Grgicevic has summarized:

The historical background is comparatively recent. The most important theory arose in 1855 when Wilhelm His named six cartilaginous hillocks as the original auricular structures. Three were formed by the mandibular arch and three by the hyoid. Other workers followed the same theory; Gradenigo (1893), Schwalbe (1877), Streeter (1992), and Gyot (1934) confirmed the six hillocks but with differences of opinion about each one. Wood-Jones and Wen I Chuan (1934) analyzed the Peking Union Medical College Collection, and found it difficult to delimit the six hillocks histologically, but observed an image near the hyoid that approached the mandibular arch and produced more than one third of the auricle, while the tragus and anterior external auricular canal appear to be the only mandibular derivatives.

The truth of His's original embryonic interpretation becomes evident in the microtic dysgenesis of the first and second arch distribution in a 6-year-old boy and in another older boy (Fig. 57).

J. Davis (1987) has observed these hillocks and related them to dysgenesis and clinical dysmorphia. In 1976 reference was made to independent periauricular perichondrium, suprauricular fascia, derived from the visceral auriculocranial meso (J. Davis).

Triaxial similarity of the mesodermal systems can explain renal pathology associated with auricular dysmorphia (A. Ferrer Rodriguez, 1979).

---

*Grgicevic was granted: FIRST PRIZE FOR "Embriología de los Arcos Branquiales" (Branchial Arch Embryology) at the Anatomy Association Congress, Argentina, 1992, and FIRST PRIZE for his work in "Sectorización de la Oreja" (Auricle sectorization), Annual Congress for Plastic and Reconstructive Surgery, Argentina, 1992.

Figure 57

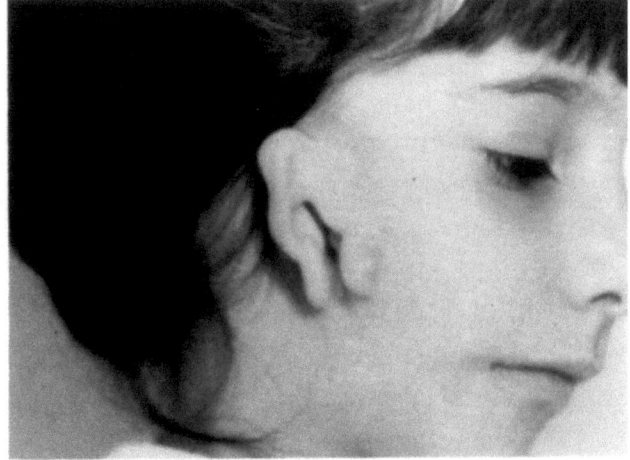
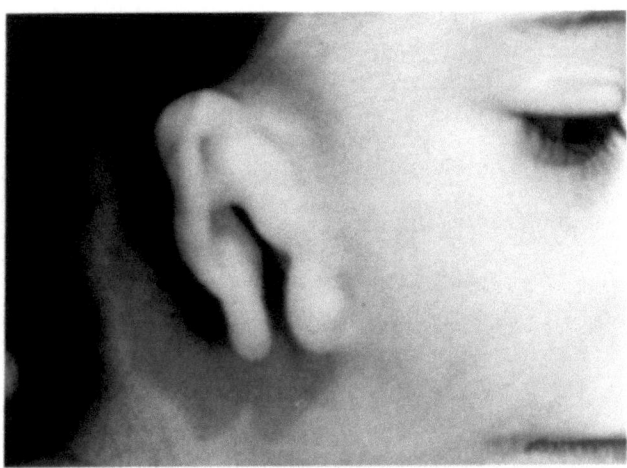
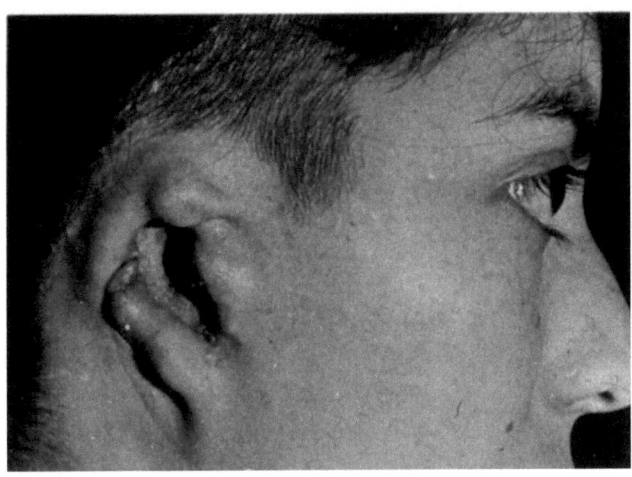

Analysis of Branchial Apparatus Concepts

In aquatic animals (fish and amphibian larvae) the gaseous interchange with blood and water occurs through the branchia, which technically act as an alveolo-ectodermal membrane. The branchia are sustained by the cartilaginous support of the branchial arches as primitive respiratory and digestive activity.

During the fourth week, the human embryo has a cranium like a fish, and develops a branchial apparatus. It is possible to infer that this branchial apparatus was originally respiratory for gaseous interchange. Anatomically, the branchial apparatus can be observed as sulci on the embryo dorsum that progress toward the anterior midline and are composed of:

1. mesodermal cartilaginous structure of the branchial arch
2. endodermal mucosa from the pharyngeal pouch
3. epidermal ectodermal structure from the branchial sulci
4. conjoined two-layer ecto-endodermal branchial membrane (mucoepidermis).

The *branchial arches* appear in the fourth week (26.3 days average) and are derived from mesodermal neural crest cells, covered by ecto- and endoderm. About 4 days later, these cells migrate and become the "branchial arches." Noden (1980) established that these neural crest cells have an ectodermal origin, but supply the mesodermic mesenchymal cranium base support.

A branchial arch forms a segment, and has a nerve derived from the neuroectoderm, an arterial and venous component, a specific cartilaginous portion, a muscular element, and therefore a specific function.

The *pharyngeal pouches* form when the primitive cranial pharynx opens superficially through the stomodeum (primitive mouth). The pharyngeal pouch endodermis covers the deep branchial arch surface forming diverticuli, specifically the pharyngeal pouches that develop between contiguous branchial arches.

The *pharyngeal membranes* are formed when the endodermal pharyngeal mucosa meets the pharyngeal epidermis. They are transitory and double-layered.

The *pharyngeal sulci* are pharyngeal grooves that separate the branchial arches, and derive from the primitive pharynx.

Embryo Organic Derivatives

From the First Branchial Arch

1. Meckel's cartilage appears at the cranial base and becomes localized behind and above the cranium, thus being enclosed by the otic capsule (formed from the otic placode). Meckel's cartilage ossifies, forming parts of the malleus, incus, lower sphenoid spine, and the pterygoid process base. The midcartilage involutions and the perichondrium form the anterior malleus ligament and sphenomaxillary ligament. The anterior part does not ossify, but contributes to the intramembranous ossification of the mandible.
2. The muscular component of the first arch is composed of the myohyoid, anterior digastric, malleous muscle, tensor velus palatinus, and the deep fascicle of the auricularis anticus. All these muscles have masticating function, and are supplied by the masticatory ramus of the trigeminal nerve.

3. When the first pharyngeal pouch is formed, it extends to the mastoid antrum and the mastoid cavity, and the distal pharyngeal mucosa lies alongside the first branchial groove endodermal mucosa, thus forming the tympanic membrane.
4. The vascular component of the first arch is formed by internal maxillary arches, derived from the external carotid.

From the Second Branchial Arch

1. Reichert's cartilage grows at the dorsal extreme of the neurocranium, but remains trapped by the otic capsule. Endochondral ossification forms the stapes and styloid process (Fig. 58). The middle third does not ossify. The perichondrium forms the stylohyoid ligament, while the anterior third creates the hyoid body and processes by intramembranous ossification.
2. The muscular components of the second arch include the group of muscles of expression, and of the stapes, stapediohyoid, and posterior digastric, which are related to mastication and partial ventilation.
3. The stapedial artery supplies the second arch.
4. Endodermis proliferation of the pharyngeal pouch forms the lymphoid crypts along the palatine section of Waldeyer's circle by 20 weeks.

Figure 58

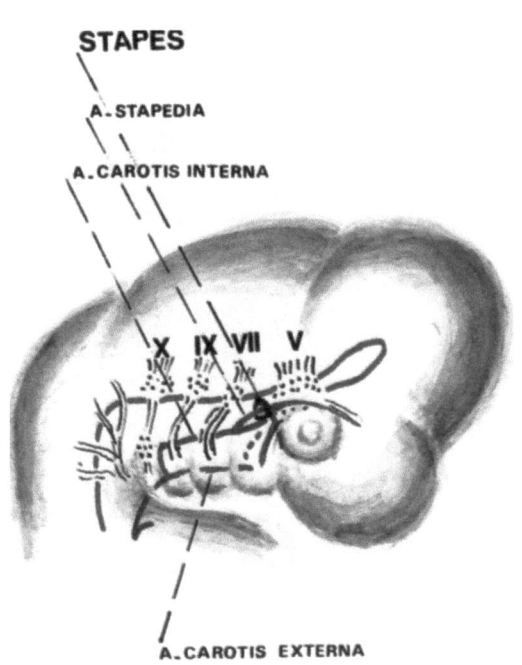

10 mm. 30 d. embryo

The Stapedial Artery

During the somatic period the arterial system has a trunk (saccus aorticus) located in front of the pharynx and has two rami that develop within the first and second arches. This period has been called "branchial circulation."

The first arch is supplied by the stapedial artery, including the mandibular arch, contents of the orbital cell, and area meningeal formation. The mandibular artery has been called the "stapes" artery by O. Llorca, with three rami: (1) supraorbitalis, which follows the ophthalmic branch of Willis of the trigeminal nerve; (2) infraorbitalis, which follows the inferior maxillary branch of the trigeminal nerve; and (3) mandibularis, which follows the maxillomandibular nerve. The artery goes through both stapedial bone rami, irrigating them, and through the perivascular membranous adventitia, and contributes to the stapes plaque cartilage formation. This system is normal until the embryo is 37 days old (17 mm). The "postbranchial circulation" appears then and lasts about 14 days. The sixth right arch and the descending right aorta disappear. During this time the stapedial artery, which originates with the internal carotid system, becomes anastomosed with the external carotid via the terminal maxillary branch. The flow becomes inverted, and the supply passes from the internal carotid, which now is named the internal maxillary artery. Defective stapedial artery supply can explain segmental congenital defects of the first arch.

Cranial Development

The skeletal system originates in the mesoderm (Fig. 59). The neural tube forms the notochord, the cartilage that governs the axial direction of embryonic growth as a cord. All vertebrae are notochords. The paraxial meso-

Figure 59

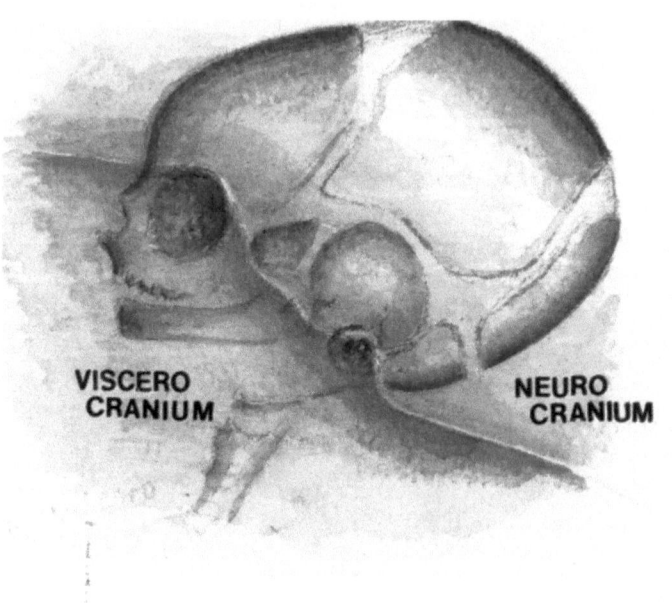

5 m. fetus

derm also becomes segmented in short lateral bodies, the somites. Each one has the following:

medially—sclerotoma, forming vertebra and ribs;

externally—myotoma, forming the muscle group;

posteriorly—dermatoma, forming the cutaneous dermis.

The mesoderm is a totipotential mesenchyma that in part originates from the neural crest and migrates toward the branchial arches. Initially bone and cartilage are mesenchymal cell condensations that determine types of ossification:

1. intramembranous ossification—the mesenchyma forms a membrane
2. endochondral ossification—ossification of preexisting cartilage.

The cranium is developed from the mesenchyma that envelops the developing cerebrum, and is constituted by a viscero- and neurocranium.

The neurocranium forms the base of the skull, and the cartilaginous neurocranium courses through three stages: desmocranium (fibrous stage), chondrocranium (cartilaginous base), and osteocranium (ossification). The membranous neurocranium is the ossification of membranes covering the skull dome bone that are squamous or diploic from conjunctival ossification.

The cartilaginous viscerocranium produces cartilage ossification of the branchial arches. The membranous viscerocranium is the ossification only of the anterior maxillary prominence of the first branchial arch, and forms the maxilla, zygoma, temporal squama, mandibular condyle ramus, and chin.

The Tympanic Ring

The tympanic ring is a special type of bone that appears on the 42nd day (±3) developed from mesenchymal mesoderm, and therefore is part of cranium base formation. It courses through three stages of chondral ossification: (1) fibrous, (2) cartilaginous, and (3) osseous.

It is the body's most uniform bone; it changes least in size with embryogenesis and has no muscle insertions, but can tolerate tension and pressure. Reinforcements are spread into the petrous bone. It is the dividing line between the cartilaginous neurocranium and membranous viscerocranium. It has two parts:

1. The tympanic ring proper that forms three quarters and is the functional body related to the temporal bone.
2. The upper quarter circle that opens between the two terminal ends of the tympanic ring, and is not of the same histology or enzymatic makeup as the ring, and can be considered a separate structure.

J. Davis has stated that the bone bordering the segment of Rivinus is in reality two different bone formations, and that each has different properties. Trophic SMAS is related to the ring, but not to adjacent bone, which is called tympanic bone. The tympanic ring does not normally form part of the external auricular canal roof that becomes adapted with later pneumatization. Defective tympanic bone–SMAS extended to the upper auricle can probably explain the "pinna–partial canal" (PPC) syndrome of Davis. Tympanic bone is ossification of the external auricular canal cartilage, and is very variable. It can be found anywhere in the canal, but when enlarged in the roof is precisely observed in the PPC syndrome. The external auricular canal cartilage advances to the tragus, which has a fibrocartilage formation, in contrast to the elastic cartilage found in the rest of the auricle. Variations of the external auricular canal are in keeping with variations of the dividing line between the neuro- and viscerocranium.

The auricle, as an auditory viscera, appears on the 24th to 25th day (± 2) with the cartilaginous hillocks around the first branchial cleft—three with the first branchial arch (mandibular or trigeminal arch) and three with the second (hyoid or facial arch). They are joined by parietal perichondrium to form the auricle and the tragus. The auricular complex first forms in the cervical area and later becomes displaced up with cranial elongation. The exact position of lobular origin has not been defined yet, but it appears at about 3 months, entirely in the cervical section.

The external auditory canal is developed at the extreme dorsum of the sulcus of the first branchial arch, which is funnel-shaped in the temporal bone. The ectodermal cells at the extreme depth of the primitive canal multiply, forming a plug that shapes the superior hemicircumference of the canal, finally shaping the external auditory canal. The mucus mesodermic plug is absorbed due to ischemia of the sinciciolisines of the respiratory substance.

The alteration of this "waterfall" mechanism produces the atresic plaque. Three examples of this process are shown in Figures 60, 61, and 62.

The primitive tympanum is the membrane of the first arch, and it is termed definite tympanic membrane with the penetration of the mesoderm from the periphery, from the canal mesoderm, and from the eustachian tube endoderm. Definite tympanic membrane has the following:

1. a *cutaneous layer*, without adnexa, similar to modified ectodermic mucosa.
2. a *fibrous mesodermic layer*, which does not cover the upper $\frac{2}{7}$ of the circle, or hiatus of Rivinus. This section is anatomically called the flaccid membrane of Shrapnell.
3. an *endodermic mucosa layer* of pharyngeal origin, which reaches the membrane via the eustachian tube.

The tympanic ring and the tympanic bone are of two different origins that depend on the SMAS trophic influence. They are two different formations, holding the membrane as an incomplete circle, and subject to considerable variations of cartilaginous ossification of the viscerocranium. Deformities of these two formations can coincide (total atresia) or be independent (partial atresia) and explain the formation of the *tympanic pouch* and the roof atresia.

There are two basic conclusions:

1. The *physiologic embryology* is most important; it later becomes projected into *functional anatomy*. Thus, the auricle as an organ, as a vis-

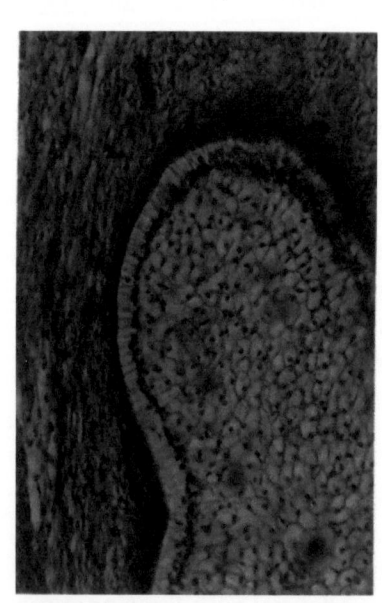

Figure 60
Section: external auricular canal of a human embryo (30 mm, 60 days). Cytolytic activity is observed with resorption of the mucose "plug."

Figure 61
Section: external auricular canal of a human embryo (23.1 mm, 50 days). The mucose plug is commencing resorption, with the appearance of polyedric basophile cells in the basal membrane, formed from the tubotympanic mesoderm.

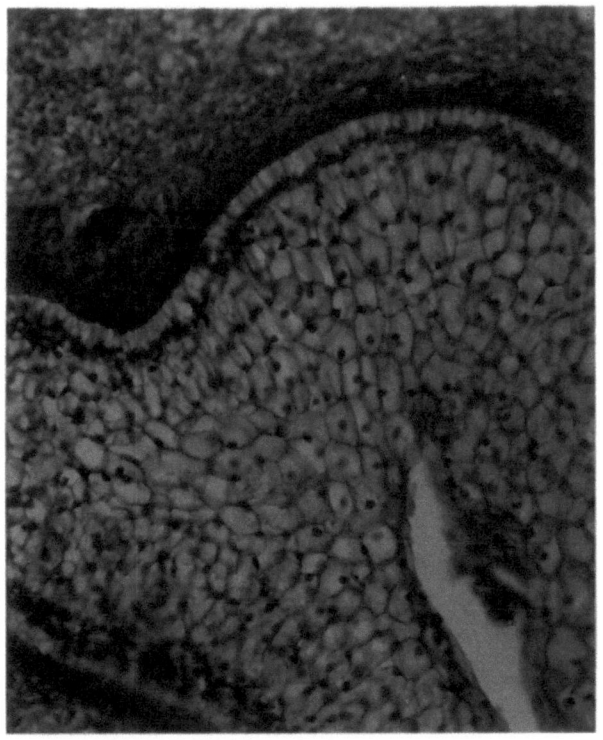

Figure 62
Section: external auricular canal of a human embryo (36 mm, 65 days). Resorption of the mucose plug, with marked changes in the basal membrane, desquamation, acidophile "lake" formation, and mesodermic fibroblastic proliferation of the middle ear.

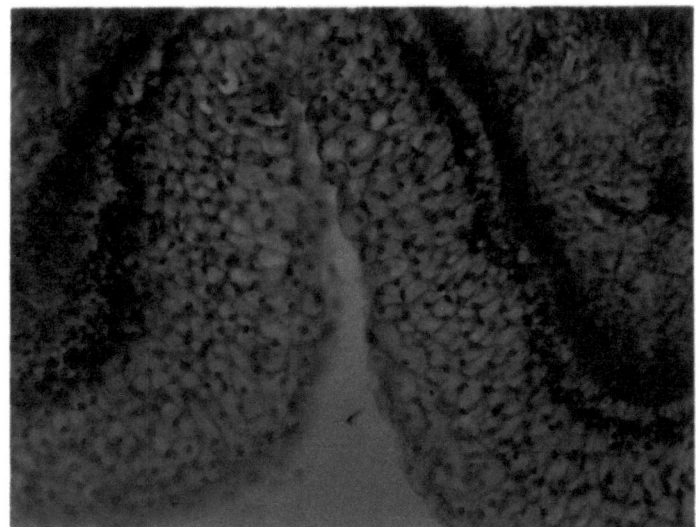

cera of a system, is considered with its functional characteristics.

2. The first and second arches plus the tubotympanic pouch are embryologically and anatomically a unit. Their deformities involve all elements of the unit, and must be considered together during clinical examination, diagnosis, and treatment.

Microtia and Auricular Atresia

It has been my privilege to have worked with an outstanding group of otosurgeons. We have shared our experiences as we labored and learned together. I particularly thank Oscar Candás (Fig. 63), Daniel Orfila, Vicente

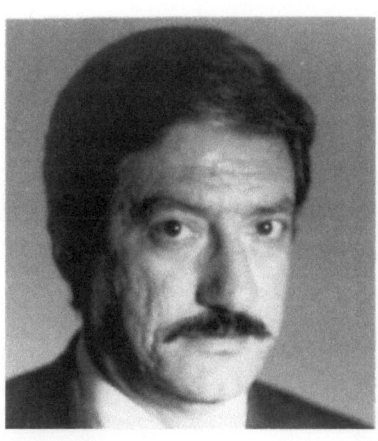

Figure 63
Dr. Oscar Candás.

Diamante, and Carlos Salvatori; they have my admiration and gratitude for our common effort.

My observations on function, and the research in embryology and cartilage by Gustavo Grgicevic, have been applied in surgery. In a relatively stagnant field, this has been a definite step forward.

We have all deeply appreciated the international work, especially by Ugo Fisch and Robert Jahrsdoerfer, that is progressing as interest grows in this subject.

On contemplating microtia-atresia repair, it is well to remember that embryologically the original mesodermic cartilage forms a substratum of basic cartilaginous formations at 21 days. At 28 days the first cartilaginous bone begins to form. From then on, both bone and cartilage change in preparation for their future functions. Thus, bone develops scaling from eburnated to cancellous to trabecular, and likewise the cartilage changes into hyaline or fibrous or elastic, each with individual characteristics in keeping with the functions they are to perform. Both bone and cartilage preserve these characteristics throughout life, and barely change when lodged in a new habitat.

Deep canal aeration does not depend on pharyngeal pneumatization at birth. When the original mesodermic cartilage in the canal area does not become transformed into bone, excess cartilage remains, and it remains undifferentiated. It does not shape a tube. The mucose plug does not form, and therefore cannot be absorbed. Fragments of cartilage may ossify, and can be seen in computed tomography (CT) scans. Abundant cartilage remains below the surface, more than that occupying the microtia, comparable to an iceberg. This atresic cartilage can indent the mastoid bone at varying depths. The surgical value is evident. Good quality and quantity of tissue is locally available. Partial differentiation of this process can explain the PPC syndrome.

The atresia is a defective formation of the canal, not a late embryonic closure.

Unilateral Microtia and Atresia

The early recognition of deformity requires studying some details carefully and methodically. Although the contralateral ear seems normal and has hearing, it has frequently been found to have minor abnormalities. It is especially important to perform early audiometric examinations on both sides, and any deficiency of the apparently sound side should be treated with hearing aids at an early age so that the child may develop normally. There is usually some difficulty with audiostereognosis with only unilateral hearing, but we have preferred to postpone CT scans until the child is 5 years old, and avoid previous x-ray exposure. High-resolution CT (HRCT) could detail the necessary information about ossicles, round and oval windows, intrapetrous facial nerve, and nerve tracts. Axial and coronal sections, with a 1-mm colimator, 3" per section, and algorithm filter for bone are used to give a three-dimensional (3D) view and to establish the distance between the surface, temporomandibular (TM) joint, and the atresic plate to plan the approach. Two points must be established: the condition of the internal ear, and detailed diagnosis of the pathology of the middle and external ears. Chronic otitis media is more frequent than expected.

Surgery is ideally done when the patient is 6 years of age; at this age the child can describe his or her deficiencies, participate in an audiometric examination, and cooperate with preoperative needs and postoperative care.

Otologic Criteria

Present otologic consideration of atresia reconstruction is a mixture of do's and dont's, what to do and what not to do. Fundamental observations include the following:

No two cases of atresia are exactly the same.

Auriculoplasty should precede otologic work.

Aggressive middle ear surgery has had the worst results.

Do not:

Attempt canal surgery without precise preoperative diagnosis (3D HRCT).

Perform posterior mastoid-antrum-attic tympanotomy.

Operate on a nonformed middle ear or one with sensorineural deafness.

Trephine a canal too narrow or too wide open.

Trephine without a neurostimulator.

Perform tympanoplastic maneuvers.

Destroy the tympanic cavity membrane.

Cover the canal with thick or hair-bearing epithelium grafts.

Do:

Preplan with HRCT, etc.

The shortest, most direct anterior approach to the atresic plate.

Trephine the canal amply enough to lodge the little finger.

Avoid nerve damage with continuous use of the stimulator.

Adequately and radically remove the atresic plate that frames and seals the surface hamulus-incus, and observe ossicle mobility and round and oval windows.

Preserve tympanic mucosa and cover it with fine, elastic sound-conducting epithelium.

Stagger canal scars.

The use of temporal fascia is still under investigation.

Should Unilateral Atresia be Operated On?

The atresic middle ear has a potential danger of otitis media complication. The only drainage is the eustachian tube. Suppuration that may follow a common cold has no safety valve outlet through soft tissue when the tube is blocked. There is no tympanic membrane to perforate, relax the pressure, and drain. Initial signs of local pain, inflammation, and fever can progress severely. The facial nerve may be affected when it is close by and exposed, due to little or no bone covering. If facial paralysis appears, the inflammation has eroded through the covering and destroyed the nerve; it is usually definitive. This can occur in a few hours, and is an indication for urgent surgery to trephine and drain, in addition to standard medical treatment. Suppurative otitis media in atresics that are not drained can abscess and spread, and cause, in order of frequency, otogenic meningitis, sinus lateralis thrombosis, and brain abscess, with early risk of death. The process can also progress as petrositis with abscess of the internal auricular canal, abscess of the cerebellum, or endolymphitis of the external semicircular canal.

Early diagnosis is imperative. The stage and localization of pus formation, and the culture-antibiotic should be established at once. The balance between medical treatment and/or type of surgery depends on the individual case, and no set rules can be established, except the urgency to stop the infection while still at its focus and before it can spread, causing these severe complications or death.

The atresic patient lives with a "time bomb" in his ear.

The other aspect of infection in the atresic is middle ear chronic disease. The process does not generally tend to spontaneous recovery, and focal or generalized inflammation can remain, due to poor eustachian tube drainage. Chronic otitis media in the atresic can produce permanent damage to the ossicular chain. The chronic inflammation can flare up anytime.

A further complication is the so-called congenital cholesteatoma. There is still much discussion about the origin, and probably there are several factors in its formation, but we have observed cholesteatoma already formed and with initial complication several times as a surgical finding; it is necessary to treat this in atresics before further damage takes place.

Cholesteatoma is observed more frequently in partial atresia, with the canal reduced to less than a 2-mm lumen. Opening the canal allows early visualization of the area, thus avoiding extensive progress of the disease.

Does the functional result justify the surgery? This depends on the severity and type of atresia, and the quality of surgery performed. In our latest series, overall average of improvement has been 25 dls., but other functions had to be considered. Audiostereognosis was close to normal, quite independently of the degree of audiometric improvement. It is difficult to measure exactly how much improvement was due to the actual surgery and how much to the patient learning to use the reconstructed organ. The psychological reaction to these changes has varied from patient to patient, but the patients' overall opinion has been that the result is satisfactory. It is necessary for the surgeon to give a clear idea of the prognosis to preclude false expectations.

Auricular Atresia

Auricular atresia has not been precisely defined. Exactly how the canal underdevelopment occurs and how the bone forms outside the middle ear has not yet been explained. Remains found along the canal tract have to be classified and detailed; this is a requirement before attempting surgery. It has been time to step ahead.

The middle and external ears have an interrelationship. Normally, there is a complementary relationship between the tympanic bone and the canal cartilage, which is embryonic, anatomic, and functional. Although there is a general relationship between the middle and external ear growth and growth abnormalities, there is a moderate independence between the tympanic cavity and the external auricular canal. There is an important relationship between the tragus and the external auricular canal, but considerably less between the tragus and the remaining auricle. The tragus embryologically forms part of the cartilage that continues with the temporomandibular joint and later mastication. The tragus is not part of the auricle; it is part of the external canal.

The canal is observed to be totally or partially closed, and therefore defined as total or partial auricular atresia.* These two categories and the way they are shaped have led us to perform an embryologic investigation, concluding that the canal is composed of two different segments: the deep juxtatympanic pouch and the superficial canal. Chronologically, the juxtatympanic pouch develops and epithelializes considerably earlier than the superficial canal segment. This interpretation considers a duplication of the tympanic bone, in which the deep tympanic bone will progress around the tympanic membrane, as an incomplete circle with a notch of Rivinus formation to form the tympanic ring, while the peripheral duplication of tympanic bone can become hypertrophied with overabundant bone superficially, which does not have a notch of Rivinus. There is a relative separation in this duplication, but there is a connection along the canal floor. This connection probably produces the continuity of the canal floor with superficial abnormalities. These findings explain the cause of *partial atresia*, which involves only the superficial segment. *Total atresia* is the underdevelopment of both deep and superficial segments.

Understanding the importance of these two canal segments is essential. The two different types of epithelium that line the canal have to be reproduced. It is imperative to obtain fine, flexible, elastic, hairless, and glandless skin over the neotympanic membrane and juxtatympanic area, but the canal meatus is preferably covered with fine flaps, downy hair, and ceruminous glands that recover the reflex defense ability.

Obtaining the necessary caliber with an even skin surface, and staggering the scars within the canal, is the surgeon's challenge and goal. This is precisely the reason for dividing auricular atresia in two—deep total and superficial partial—and projecting the embryology for adequate reconstruction.

Canal

As the private secretary tends the sanctuary of the president's inner office and knows what is going on, so does the *tragus* tend the canal and middle ear. Precisely positioned in the antechamber of sound entry, to police and

---

*Davis JE. *Aesthetic and Reconstructive Otoplasty*. New York: Springer-Verlag; 1987.

guard this entry, it is normally formed by the fusion of embryonic hillocks 6 and 1, and found at birth as the tragus proper and the tuberculum supratragicum of His, sealed as one entity.

I stress once again that any tragus abnormality is of important diagnostic value, and calls for immediate, thorough, and detailed examination of the canal and middle ear. The need for adequate anatomophysiologic canal patency for sound entry is obvious. But it is important to understand that as the canal is functionally part of the external ear, it is most definitely part of auriculoplasty.

Details of some congenital canal abnormalities have been rarely recorded in the literature. Congenital canal atresia associated with pinna dysmorphism has been previously published by this author* and therefore the following cases of severe partial atresia with poor hearing, normalized by surgery, can be enlightening.

Partial Atresia Syndromes

I have been deeply impressed by the striking similarity of a group of cases that clinically had signs and symptoms sufficient to classify them as partial auricular atresia syndromes. This led to a further investigation and studies by Gustavo Grgicevic and his group, and we were able to pattern the following embryologic, clinical, and surgical progress from our observations.

A superficial skin opening in the lower part of the concha or below the auricular area in the upper neck has been repeatedly observed. The site of this opening was always low as compared with the auricle. The size of the opening was 1 to 3 mm, with well-developed skin and with hair and ceruminous glands. On exploring the opening with a fine probe, preferably a lacrimal duct probe, it was found to continue as a fistula of the same caliber and a similar type of skin. The direction of the fistula was upward and slightly forward. At about a 12-mm depth the tip of the probe danced around in a cavity, as the fistula had expanded and widened out. There was no secretion or pus from inflammation of this deeper cavity, so the tract had been sufficient to eliminate desquamation, but cerumen blocked the passageway. The probe exploration was not continued more deeply, or blindly, for fear of traumatizing a tympanic membrane below. Further manual exploration was avoided. Microscopic vision was obscured by the cerumen blocking the lumen, and by the narrow opening. Injecting radiopaque solutions for a fistulography is awkward and uninformative. The best preoperative diagnosis is with HRCT.

This single-tract fistula should not be confused with preauricular tags, cysts, or fistula that can reach the middle ear. The preauricular formations are due to otomandibular defects of coalescence of the first arch. In contrast, this subauricular single tract fistula was a malunion of the first and second arches.

With CT scanning and later surgery, it was established that the canal was bottle-shaped and the neck opened out into a normal or nearly nor-

---

*Davis JE. *Aesthetic and Reconstructive Otoplasty*. New York: Springer-Verlag; 1987.

mal calibered canal, with a normal or nearly normal tympanic membrane. The type of skin that covered this deep canal was entirely different from the fistula. The skin was very fine, with little desquamation, no hairs or glands of ceruminous type, and minimum subcutaneous tissue. I have named this deep canal pseudocavity the juxtatympanic pouch.

The abnormal hypotresic lumen stricture was not sharply defined, but feathered off gently in every direction. The important finding was that the stricture affected the roof of the canal. It was formed of soft or hard tissue, and was quite unique. When it was formed only of soft tissue, the subcutaneous tissue had fragmented cartilage, muscle fibers, trabeculated fat, and ceruminous glands mixed up in a disorderly fashion. When the stricture was hard it was made up of a bony mass, covered by a little soft tissue. The bony mass was relatively ovoid, formed by cancellous bone with a thin surface condensation. The striking factor was that the bony mass could be dissected along a plane of coalition, from the temporal squama. The mass was tympanic bone.

The other important finding was that the fistula–juxtatympanic pouch floor was continuous and level. Although the type of skin covering of these two sections was very different, both could be well dissected to shape fine flaps, with excellent circulation and viability. The flaps were used for canal lining.

Grgicevic has stated, "What is the ontologic basis of the Davis syndrome? It is a trophic defect of the tympanic bone, but not of the tympanic ring, involving the stage of cartilaginous fibrosis of the tympanic bones that during their growth press against each other and expand towards the external auricular canal roof trophism and the upper auricle, without affecting the canal floor."

The association with the upper auricle will be described later. The surgical value of these observations is evident. The auricle and canal are reconstructed in one stage. Precision preoperative diagnosis is necessary to prepare for the bone surgery, to remove the osseous roof excess following the plane of cleavage formed by tiny remains of cartilage and fibrous tissue, and then to bur off the edges. All local skin is carefully preserved and well used, but after amplifying the canal caliber 50% to avoid secondary retraction the final defect is closed with a mastoid skin graft to complete the lining. Hearing improves radically, in keeping with the correction of conductive loss.

Case

This 13-year-old boy consulted us for a left unilateral microtia. On examining his right ear as a donor site, the bifid tragus was apparent. I went straight in to have a look at the canal, and found it subtotally blocked with hard tissue. A minimal canal of 1.7-mm lumen remained in the lower concha. The canal was patent, containing wax, and comparatively straight. The mass that blocked it was palpated and found to have some soft tissue, some cartilage, but nearly all bone. There was no inflammation or discharge. Nothing further was visualized with the microscope (Fig. 64).

Audiometry showed a 35-dB conductive loss, and CT scan showed a normal middle ear and tympanic membrane, but a superficial absence of the canal.

Figure 64

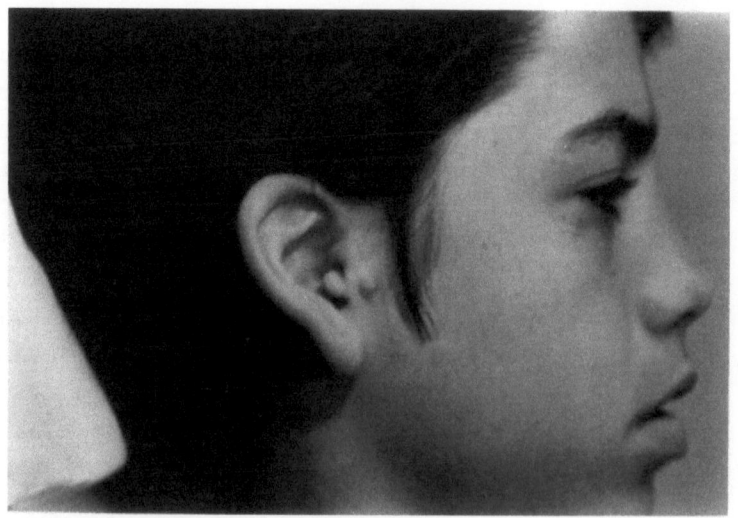

Surgery of the canal was performed simultaneously with the first stage of the contralateral microtia repair. The length of the canal had been calculated with the probe and tomographs to be 14 mm. A long vertical skin flap was outlined on the conchal floor, and then extended along the conchal roof, as shown (Fig. 65). This allowed ample exposure to the area of the mass blocking the canal. On incising the skin, fatty and fibrous tissue was found, with irregular muscle fibers and fragments of abnormal cartilage that were removed and analyzed. No pathologic tissue was found.

The canal skin was then very carefully detached from the bone with tiny middle ear elevators, until the bone was bared but the skin flaps kept intact. There was no spine of Henle or notch of Rivinus.

On starting the osteotomy, a layer of synostosis was found that seemed

Figure 65

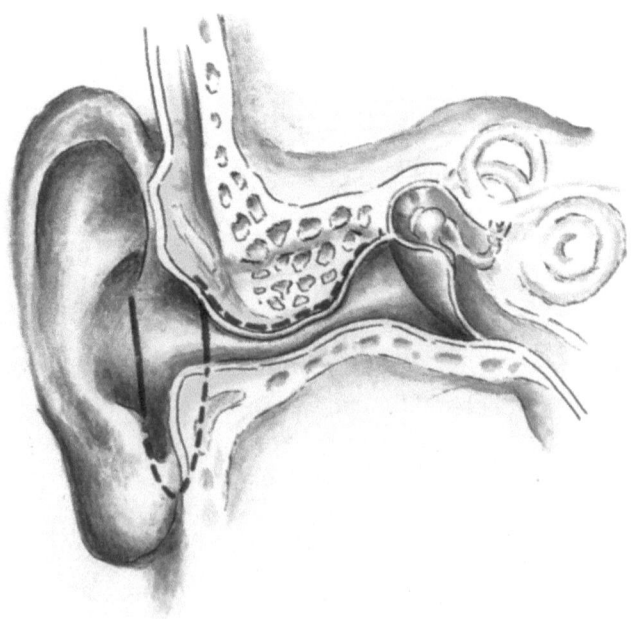

to be the union of tympanic and squamous bone. There were tiny cartilaginous fragments along this plane. Osteotomy was performed first with a sharp Freer elevator and then with a bayonet gouge chosen to fit the needed size of caliber precisely.

The bone was removed en bloc, as shown (Fig. 66). A bur was avoided because the heat would have severely affected flap and graft survival.

The narrow canal did indeed open into a pretympanic ampoule, and a large, normal tympanic membrane came into view.

The canal skin was kept to line the walls, and the long vertical conchal flap rotated up along the new canal roof, as a modified Z-plasty. The wound borders were held with a few 7-0 silk sutures, as illustrated in Figure 67, and then the canal was very lightly packed with antiseptic Vaseline wool.

The result was excellent. The neocanal progressed with normal caliber, good axial direction, smooth walls normally waxed, and a beautiful tympanic membrane was observed in the depth (Fig. 68). Hearing improved 30 dB, which was doubly important because the other side was completely atresic. Social hearing became satisfactory and practically normal. The air-bone gap was reduced to normal (Fig. 69).

The bifid tragus was also corrected to improve aesthetics, with a modified Z-plasty joining the tragus proper with the tuberculum supratragicum of His (Fig. 70).

The advantage of using these triple flaps is that they are unquestionably superior to a skin graft. Although flap work in the canal is more demanding and needs greater experience to calculate viability, sudoriparous and sebaceous glands provide the necessary humidity and cerumen, and downy hairs supply spontaneous cleaning. The texture is the closest to canal skin, and there is primary sensation and trophism. Less fibrous tissue will

Figure 66

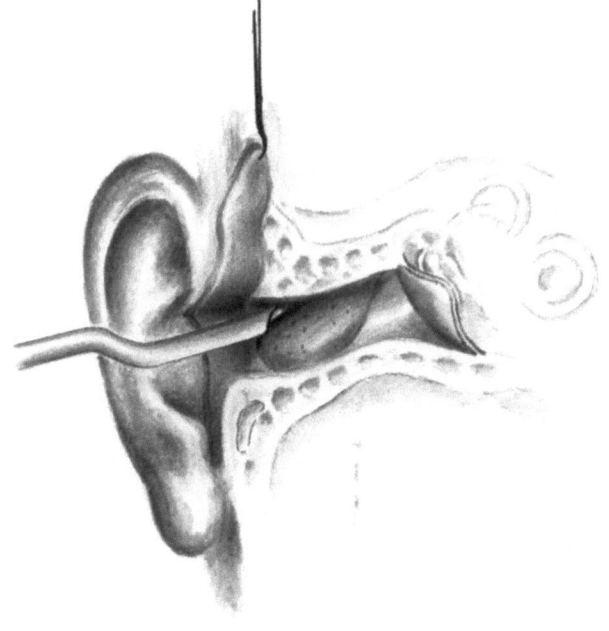

Figure 67

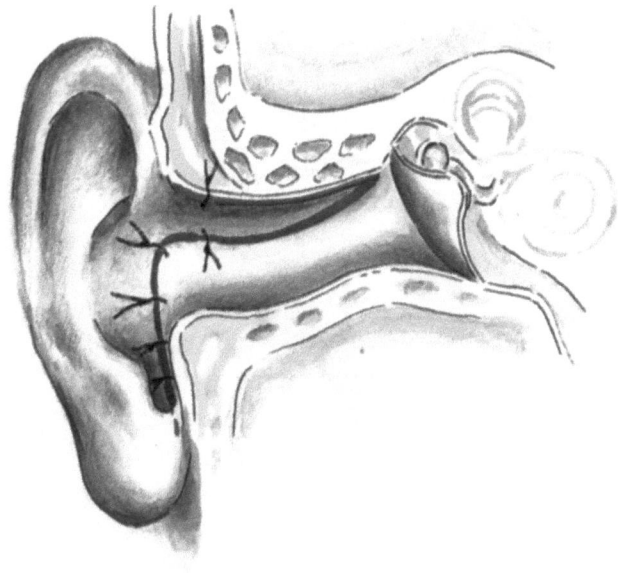

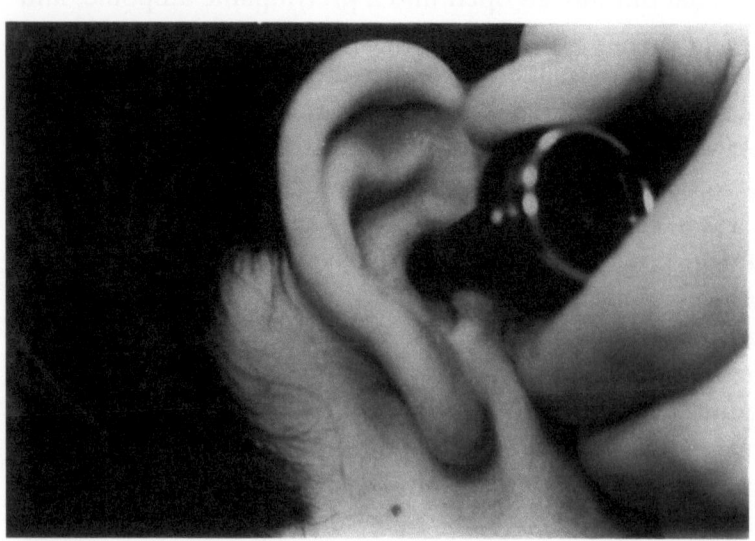
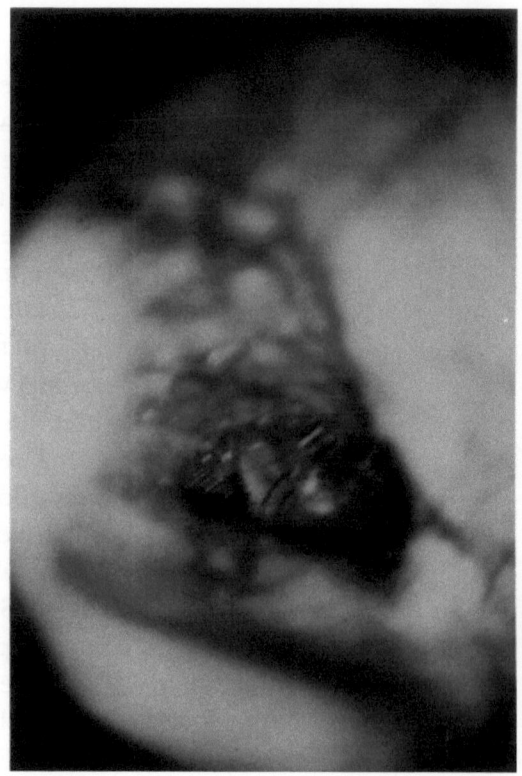

Figure 68

form under these flaps, contributing to surface softness and pliability. The scars are finally minimal and do not stenose the canal. The flap is more resistant to infection and has better healing potential. The patency during the early postoperative course will contribute to the flap's de-swelling, and the canal caliber will increase for 1 year after surgery.

In contrast, thin split-thickness grafts "take" easier. They have been usually removed from the hairless medial arm aspect as a donor site. The "take" takes 5 days, but for several weeks there is considerable desquamation. Desquamation plus purulent discharge should not be confused with wax. Once healed, the skin grafts were very rigid, because of the abundant fibrous tissue that formed under them. The skin grafts, fibrous bed, and

Figure 69

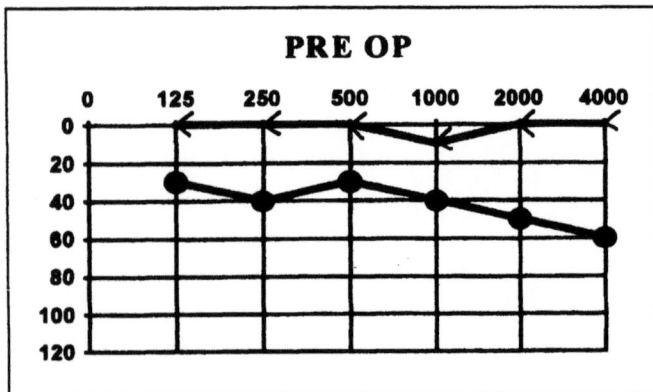
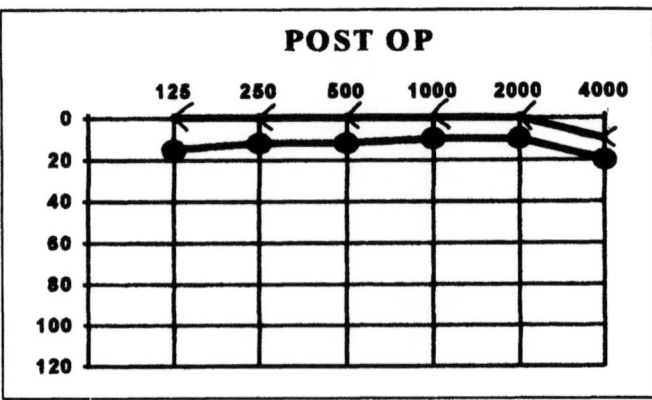

Chapter Three **Moderate Microtia and Partial Atresia**

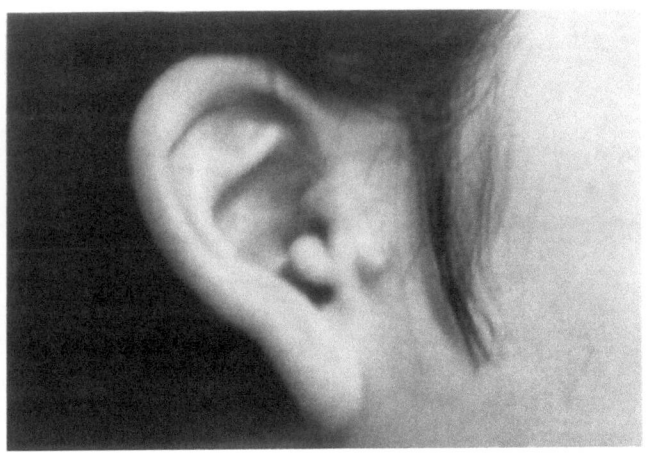
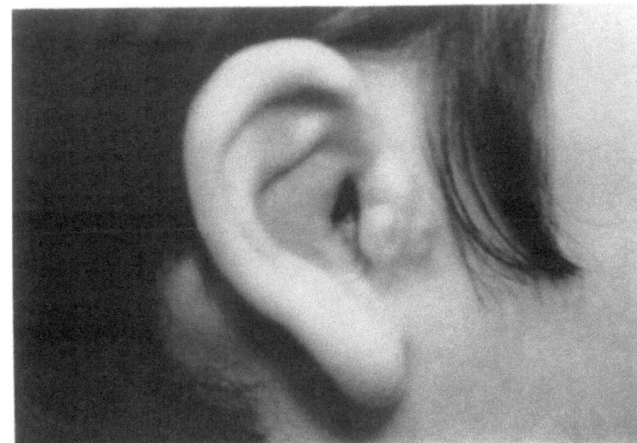

Figure 70
Pre and Post

scars contracted considerably. The worst contractures were circular, especially when the circle was the canal tube perimeter. The measure of contracture could not be preestablished, and varied from patient to patient. The thinner skin grafts produced more contracture. Thus, a 50% excess canal opening has been allowed, to calculate for these contractures. Once the contractures had produced stenosis of the canal, pretended moulded expanders have proved useless. Resistance to infection was lower than with flaps, and healing potential also was lower. Recovery of sensation was nearly nil. Fortunately, to my knowledge keloids have not been observed in the neocanals, but they have been observed in the adjacent auricular reconstruction.

An important factor for good skin graft "take" in the canals has been the correct pressure upon it, which has to be maintained at least 5 days. When simultaneous grafts and flaps were used together, it was imperative that the flaps received minimal pressure upon them. The pressure balance has been exacting. Although the medial arm split-skin graft has been commonly used, I think that the best for canal reconstruction is very thin full-thickness skin, taken from the upper eyelid or prepuce. These grafts have been fine, elastic, mobile, and well vascularized. They have to be very precisely prepared, placed and covered with nonadhesive, before applying mild pressure on them for 6 days. Penis foreskin in dark-skinned people can become deeply pigmented for 4 years, and then pale.

It has been necessary to care for the canal at least during the first 2 years, and longer when grafts were used. Repeated cleaning with soap and peroxide is necessary, syringed and rinsed out with tepid water. Antiseptics should be avoided; they are caustic and can easily harm the delicate new surfaces.

This abnormality was interpreted as an excessive formation of tympanic bone. The concept of duplication of the tympanic bone has been expressed previously, one covering the canal and the other shaping the annulus tympanicus (tympanic ring) around the membrane. The anterior and posterior tympanic bone tubercula, which were long and large, pressed against

Figure 71

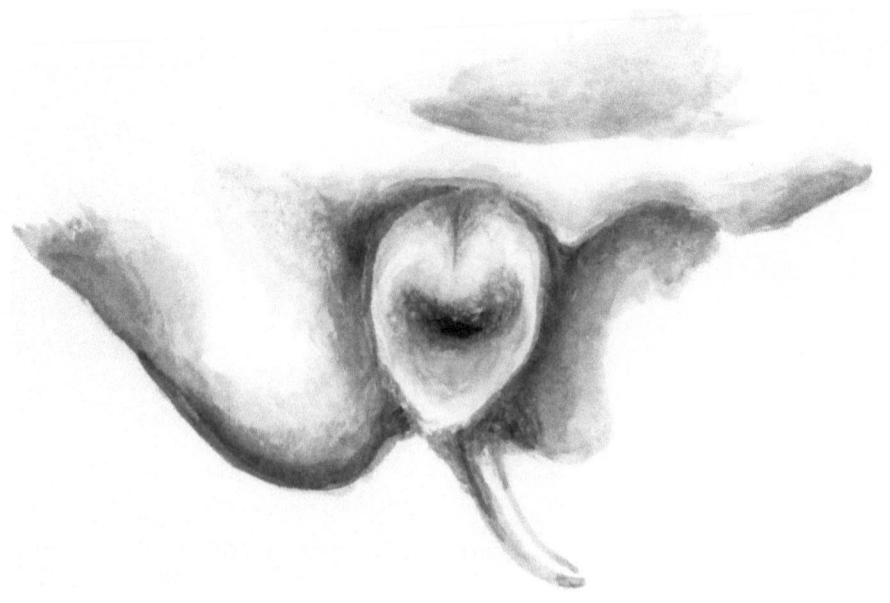

each other with growth, and as they progressed superficially, curled inward the external auricular canal lumen, and later synostosed together. Therefore, a line of demarcation indicated the division between the tympanic bone and the temporal squama, which marked the pathway for osteotomy, as shown in Figure 71.

4 The Cartilage

During our surgery we have observed that hyaline (costal) cartilage grafted into the auricular area did not become integrated into its new habitat, but formed a pseudocapsule around it. This fibrous pseudocapsule was not a bridge for new vessels and nerves penetrating into the graft, but rather a layer of bed tolerance. No capillaries or nerves were seen in the graft. Imbibition was minimal. The pseudocapsule was easily peeled away from the chondrograft, without bleeding. Hematomata formation occurred between the pseudocapsule and the graft. The graft trophism was not normal. Growth was erratic and unpredictable. In its new media, the graft aged quickly, became rigid, hard as wood, and then calcified. It did not acquire sensation as the normal side. It did not have movement, nor form a part of facial expression. Resistance to trauma and infection was poor. The graft became isolated, without normal biologic relationship with its neighboring tissues. It did not function as part of the first and second arches, nor comply with all the functional auricular characteristics.

Therefore, although shape and color could be good, costal (hyaline) cartilage in the auricular area was never really part of the patient. Above all, it blocked the otosurgeon's best approach to the middle ear, leaving only the retroauricular mastoid access to the tympanic cavity.

In contrast, elastic (auricular) cartilage became incorporated in every sense when grafted into the auricular area; it showed delicacy, flexibility, elasticity, revascularization, and innervation, with normal trophism and growth and without capsular formation. The perichondrium was observed as a bridge for capillaries and nerves, which incorporated the graft intimately with its surrounding tissues. SMAS gave movement as part of facial expression. The auricle became pale and congested with emotion and temperature changes. Sensation became symmetrical with the normal side. Healing potential was normal and equal to the other ear. Children could practice martial arts or high dive. They could have their ears pulled on birthdays. They could pull a turtleneck jersey over their heads without the ear catching in the wool. The flexibility and elasticity permitted the use of eyeglass earpieces. The door was opened for the otosurgeon to reach the middle ear by the anterior approach, shorter and directly to the hamulus and atresic plate.

These clearly defined clinical and surgical observations need explanation and research to establish why these variations took place.

Basic Considerations

Skeletal tissue, be it bone or cartilage, is essentially specialized connective tissue, formed by (1) cells, (2) intercellular matrix, and (3) fibrillar system. Physically, the tissues differ due to their solidified matrix. Phylogenetically, cartilage is an ancient tissue, found in all vertebrates. In humans, during embryonic development the skeleton is only cartilage that becomes ossified in some areas. Cartilage remains, however, in the articular surfaces, thorax, bronchi, nose, eyelids, and ears. Cartilage characteristics include low metabolic level and vascularization, interstitial and appositional growth capacity, and high resistance to traction and compression. The cartilage cells are called chondrocytes. The intercellular matrix varies according to the specific function with which they must comply. They are classified as follows:

1. Hyaline cartilage (*hyalos* means glass)
2. White fibrocartilage (contains collagen)
3. Yellow elastic cartilage (contains an elastine network).

The cartilage cells fill small lacunar spaces in the matrix. Young cells, called chondroblasts, are relatively small and flat and have an irregular edge with pseudopodic-type extensions lodged in the matrix. Postmitotic chondroblasts have intercellular contact and are absorbed with matrix synthesis. The chondrocytes are mature cells that grow and become spheroid with age and lose the extensions.

The matrix is composed chiefly of water, proteoglycans, lipids, and collagens. The substance is a firm gel, positive to periodic acid-Schiff reaction, and metachromatically to toluidine blue. The glycoproteins are a series of mucoprotein copolymers, conjoined in large lateral chains without rami, of condroitin-4-sulfate glycosaminoglycans, condroitin-6-sulfate, and keratan sulfate. The proportions are modified with age; keratan sulfate increases. The condroitin-4-sulfate and the condroitin-6-sulfate are formed by the production of N-acetylgalactosamine and glucuronic sulfate, differing only with the position of the sulfate ester. The acidity of these polysaccharide sulfates causes the basophilia, metachromatism, selective permeability, and viscoelastic characteristics of the matrix.

The collagen is different from that found in other vertebrates. The human tropocollagen is composed of three chains of alpha-1, which are identical. The resistance to compression and the viscoelasticity of the cartilage are due to their content in glycosaminoglycans, and the resistance to tension of the collagen content.

Nutrition

Cartilage has been described as an avascular tissue, because the vessels are so far away from the cells. Vascularity reaches the perichondrium membrane at the cartilage block surface. Nutrient substances and metabolite interchange pass from the perichondrial capillaries to the chondrocytes by diffusion, following a concentration gradient through the matrix. Nutrition is through the cartilage canals, which contain a few small vessels that branch from a perichondrial artery and vein. The vessels end in the canal's fundus, with some capillaries. These vessels are in lax connective tissue, with fibroblasts and macrophages connected to the perichondrium. Canal formation is produced by chondrolysis, when the chondrocytes leave the canals, and are destroyed by anoxia. The canals are distributed in the cartilage mass they must supply, and are related to the formation of secondary condensation centers. This process of supply is present in the auricular cartilage throughout life, as are others derived from the first and second branchial arches. The perichondrium is important because it is supplied by a visceral layer, as defined by Davis, as it is trophic and has a parietal layer of secondary supply.

Varieties

Hyaline Cartilage

Hyaline cartilage has a pearly blue appearance, is translucent and homogeneous, of a firm consistency, with spheroid or polygonal cells, distributed in groups of two or more cells produced from a common "mother." These groups are called nests. The matrix is typically basophile, with a metachromic reaction, which is most pronounced when recently formed matrix constitutes the periphery of a lake containing cells. The different areas are called territorial matrix or lacunar capsule in contrast to interterritorial matrix, which stains poorly. When the matrix is observed, it seems transparent, but does not have a structure similar to glass. When seen with polarized light, it has a system of fibers and fibrils, of 10 to 20 nm in diameter, with the characteristic band of 64 nm of collagen. It has permanent autogenous chondrolysis, and ossifies with age from osteoid reaction with calcium deposits in the lacunar formations. In costal cartilage, the cells and nuclei are large, and the matrix is homogeneous and has a fibrous striation that becomes accentuated with age. Large vascular canals can be seen, and eventually medullary elements, and quantitative studies have demonstrated a reduction of cellularity in all costal cartilage, thus reducing its resistance and increasing its fragility.

Fibrous Cartilage

Fibrous white cartilage is dense tissue, distributed with fibers and small groups of cells between the fibers, surrounding concentric and striated areas of cartilaginous matrix. The auricular bone surfaces are covered with white fibrocartilage. The deeper layers adjacent to bone are calcified, hypertrophic, and degenerated in areas around articular hyaline cartilage. The superficial layer is composed of parallel groups of fibers of collagen, intermixed with fibroblasts that are typical of connective tissue with little fundamental substance.

Elastic Cartilage

Elastic yellow cartilage is found in the auricle and some branchial derivatives. It contains typical chondrocytes, but the matrix has a network of yellow elastic fibers, except at the lake borders. The fibers are resistant to acetic acid, have affinity with orcein, and do not have the periodicity observed with the electron microscope. The histogenesis of the elastic fibers is in two stages: first, a microfibrillar network of oxytalan glycoprotein, and second, impregnation with elastine. It is particularly important to note that elastic cartilage has vibratory properties, which are fundamental for sound wave reception.

Histogenesis, Growth, and Regeneration

Cartilage is formed initially from embryonic mesenchyma. The mesenchyma condenses; that is, the cells multiply and group together, creating the cartilage mass. The cells have irregular surface projections with the condensing mesenchyma, and are covered with a fine basophilic layer composed of a fine network of associated collagen and chondromucoprotein filaments, which are secreted by the cells. The original cells become chondroblasts, each in a primitive cartilaginous lake. The secretion continues, and fibers and matrix are separated from the cells until mature cartilage is formed.

Interstitial Growth

The mitotic division continues, and the primitive chondroblasts are condensed in the cartilage mass. When a cell divides, the "children" occupy the same lake, but soon the cells become separated, and with the subdivisions produce an isogenous group.

Appositional Growth

Cell proliferation continues in the deeper perichondrial layers. Some of the cells, however, remain on the cartilage surface, becoming chondroblasts that secrete a matrix layer, and are included in superficial lakes. This process produces a surface increase, which is the appositional growth.

Regeneration

Cartilage capacity to regenerate lost tissue is limited. The defect is filled slowly with connective granulation tissue that can become devascularized and persist a long time as fibrous tissue.

Normal cartilage growth depends on adequate nutritional substratum and hormone balance. It has little matrix antigenicity, poor vascularization, and chondrocyte isolation in lakes.

With these observations, we should define the behavior of hyaline and elastic cartilage more precisely, from a surgical viewpoint, so further investigation is necessary.

Investigation

An investigation was performed by Gustavo Grgicevic (Fig. 72), grafting rabbit cartilage, rib-to-ear costal cartilage (CC), and ear-to-ear auricular cartilage (AC) (Fig. 73). Grafting was done with microdissection. Specimens were removed at 120 days, which would correspond to about 3.3 years in

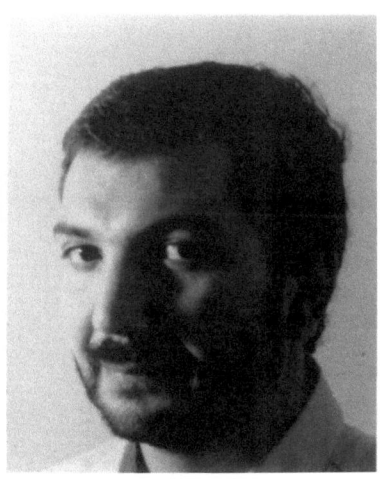

Figure 72
Dr. Gustavo Grgicevic

the human life span. The investigation involved 38 grafts. Inclusion was in Epon block 128. Sections were ultrafine. Coloration varied and is detailed in the following examination. Observations were done with high-resolution light microscopy (HRLM).

The following figures illustrate the method used, approaching the dorsal ear aspect and placing autogenous auricular and costal cartilage grafts in the rabbit ear. Figures 74 and 75 show the removal and introduction into the recipient site of auricular cartilage, and Figures 76 and 77 show the same for costal cartilage. The surgeon, technique, and conditions were the same in all animals. A few sections have been selected to show the results observed (Figs. 78–92).

The remainder of the histopathologic examination was routine. The material was prefixed with 3% glutaraldehyde in a buffer suspension of sodium cacodylate (0.1 mol/L). It was included in Polibed R.

The specimens were sectioned with 1-μm thickness. Staining was principally with toluidine blue and fuscin for HRLM, and acetate uranile-Reynolds for electron ultramicroscopy.

The previous cases for which HRLM was performed and the following electronic ultramicroscopy cases were managed by Gustavo Grgicevic with the assistance of Nestor Ruben Lagos, Director of the Laboratory of Experimental Pathology, Department of Pathology, Buenos Aires University, under conditions and controls in keeping with medical research programs.

The electronic ultramicroscopy findings have confirmed the HRLM investigation, and served to dispel any doubts about chondrocyte behavior. The difference between AC and CC is apparent, and the following electronic microscopy examples (Figs. 93 to 96) are shown to illustrate CC degeneration.

Figure 73

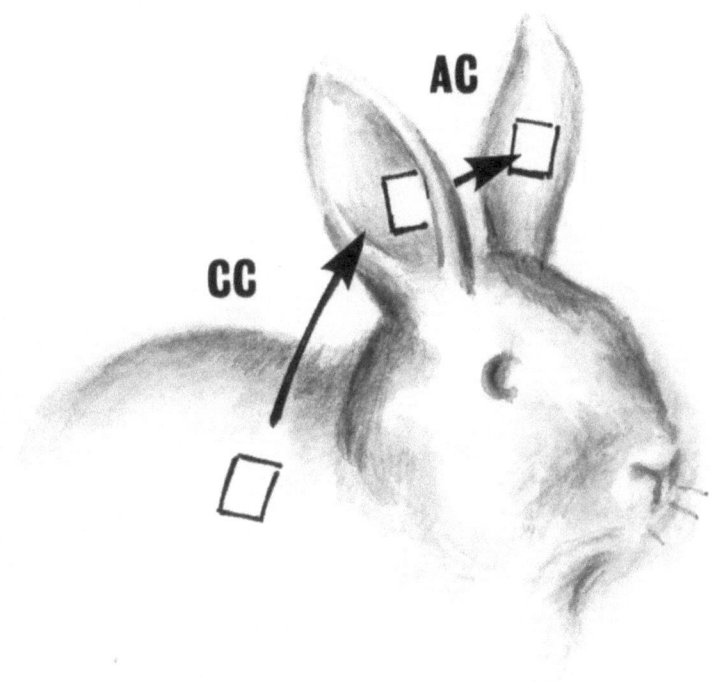

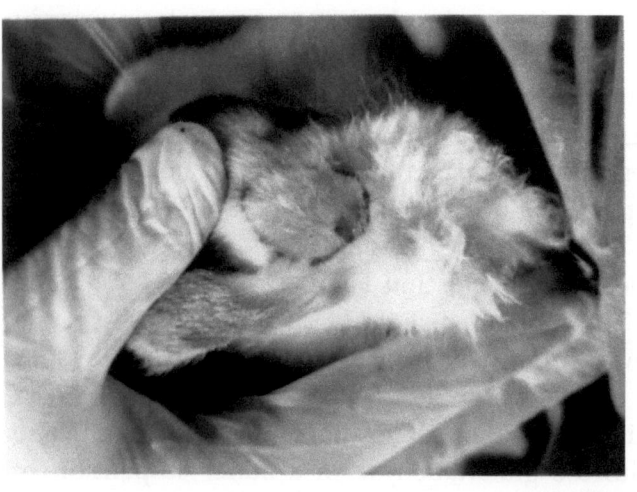
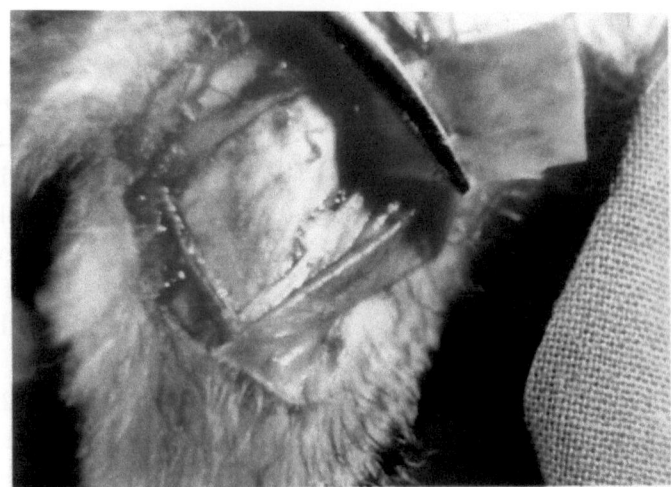

Figure 74

Figure 75

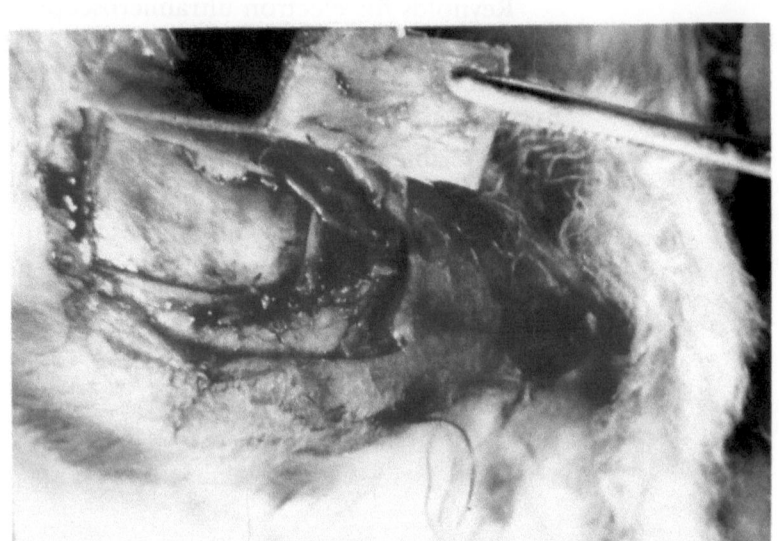

Figure 76

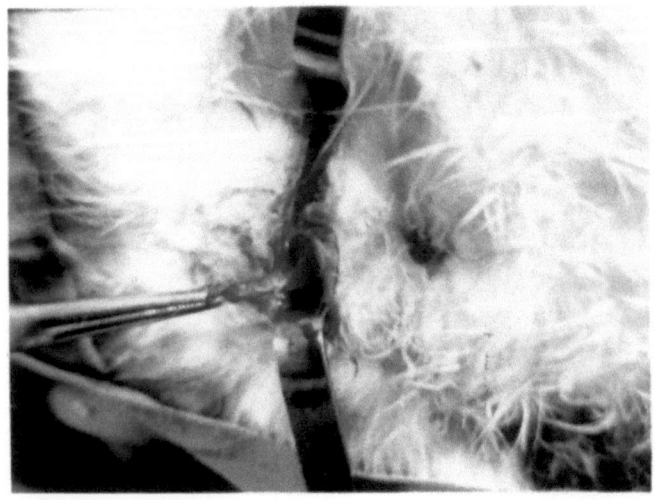
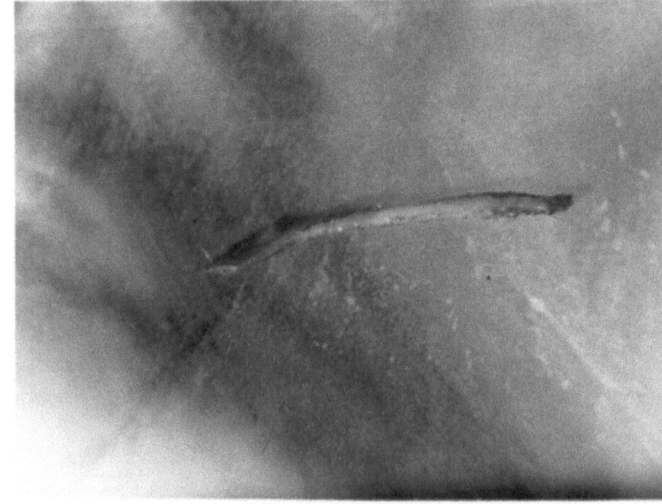

Chapter Four **The Cartilage**

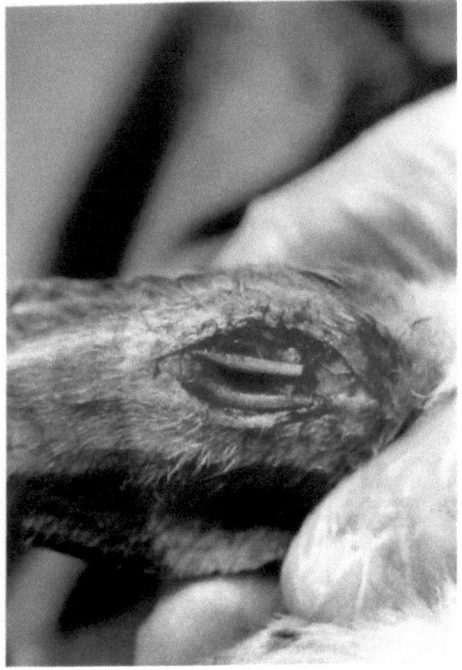

Figure 77

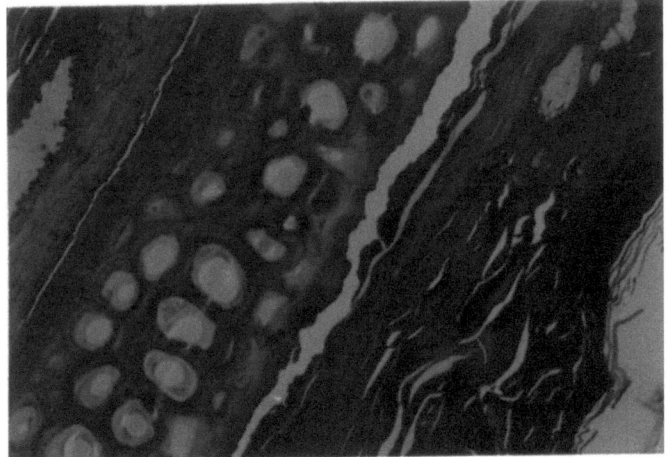

Figure 79
AC rabbit. 120 days PO. Toluidine fuscin stain. ×250 (HRLM). The following observations were reported: preserved chondrocyte viability, without subjacent collagen reaction; in the upper left area an artery has no perivascular fibrosis.

Figure 80
AC rabbit. 120 days PO. Toluidine fuscin stain. ×275 magnification (HRLM). The pseudocapsule is seen, and within it a trophic nerve with an artery that reaches the SMAS. Polygonal muscle fibers are preserved, with acidophilic cytoplasm and an acidophilic intermyofibrillar net of the subsarcolemmal nuclei. Grafted chondrocyte activity is trophic, homogeneous, and integrated with the underlying muscle.

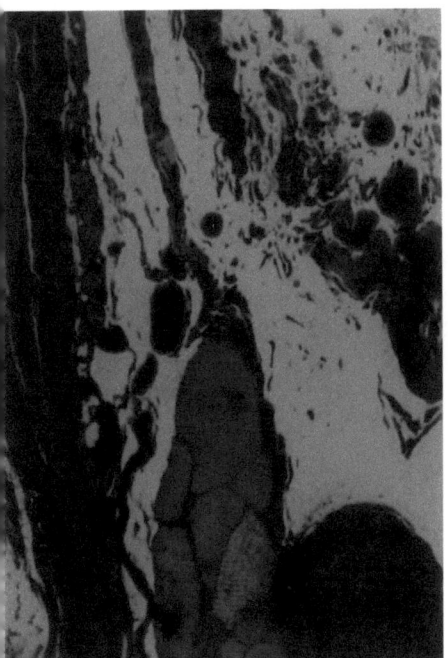

Figure 78
AC rabbit. 120 days postoperative (PO). Toluidine fuscin stain. ×125 magnification (HRLM). Preserved muscle striations were observed. Normally trophic SMAS. No fibrous reaction.

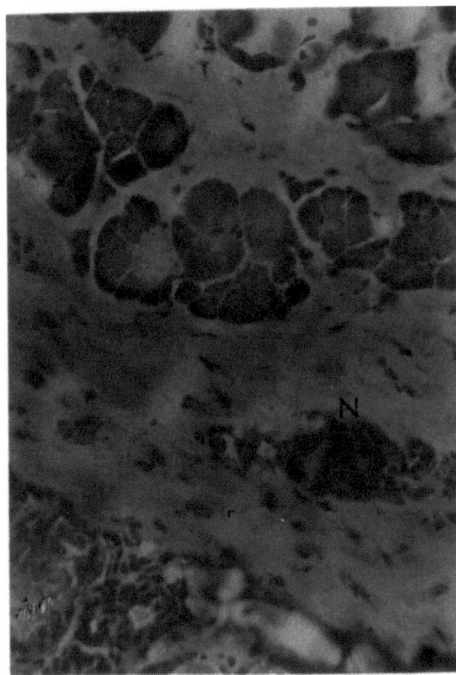

Figure 81
AC rabbit. 120 days PO. Toluidine fuscin stain. ×400 magnification (HRLM). Trophic vessels are observed in the pseudocapsule. Normal chondrocyte activity and trophism.

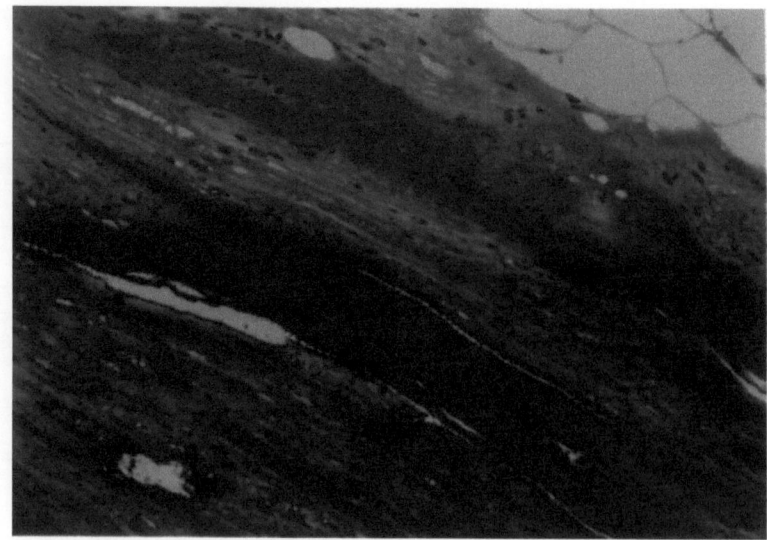

Figure 82
AC rabbit. 120 days PO. Specimen fixed with 2.5% glutaraldehyde at 4°C, and with 10% formaldehyde. Osmium tetraoxide stain. Sectioned at 5-μm thickness. ×125 magnification (HRLM). Major nerve fasciculi are observed, joined by epineurial connective tissue of dense collagen of cylindroid type. The epineurium carries vasa vasorum and fibroblasts that penetrate the fibroblastic capsule surrounding the graft, as a neurovascular bundle that supplies the isogenic groups of chondrocytes and aids muscular striation.

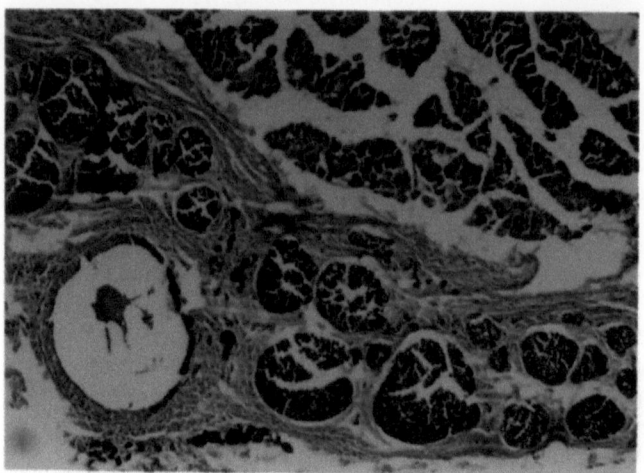

Figure 83
CC rabbit. 120 days PO. Toluidine fuscin stain. ×50 magnification (HRLM). Observations reported: Necrotic areas, due to histic anoxia. Fibrous pseudocapsule. The invasion of connective and granulation tissue, and fibrous bands (intracartilaginous fibrosis) replaces the costal cartilage graft. Resorption of the grafted costal cartilage is noted.

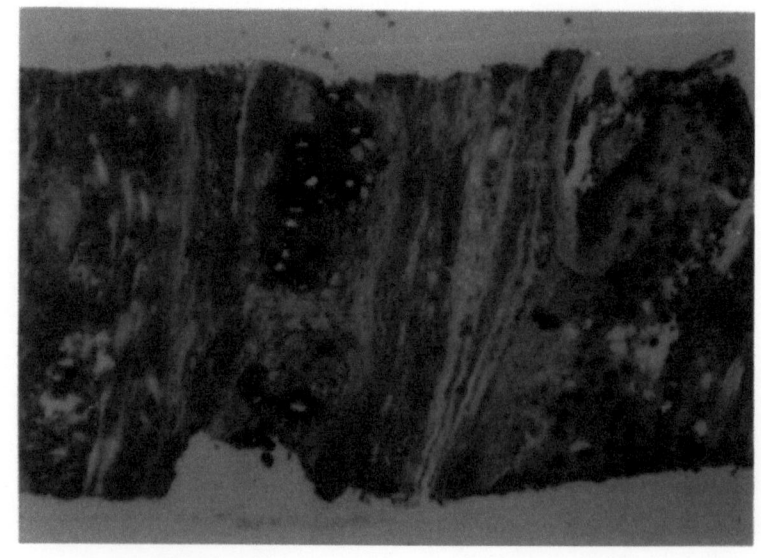

Figure 84
CC rabbit. 120 days PO. Stained with toluidine fuscin. ×100 magnification (HRLM). The pseudocapsule of the costal cartilage graft was found not to have adapted to the adjacent auricular cartilage. The pseudocapsule had bands of fibroconnective tissue, with areas of cartilage replacement by primitive fibrous tissue.

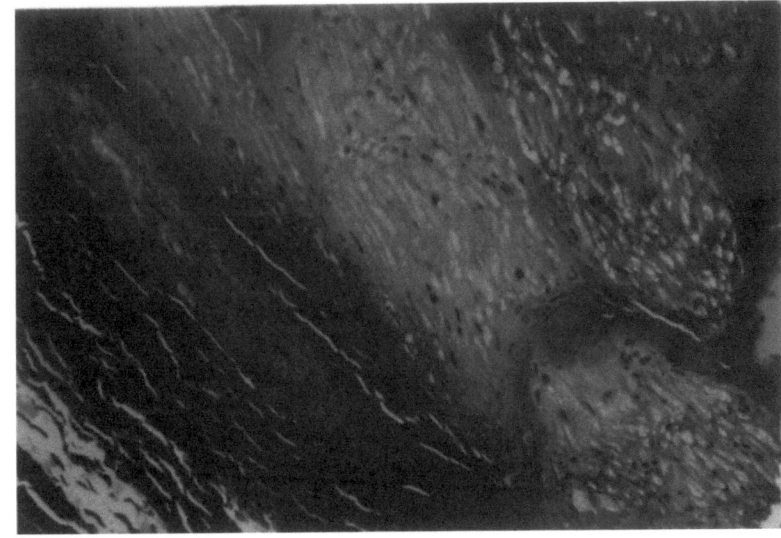

Figure 85
CC rabbit. 120 days PO. Toluidine fuscin stain. ×125 magnification (HRLM). Pseudocapsular formation is observed. SMAS is without striation. Chondrocytes are in the degenerative stage. Perivascular hyalinosis is noted.

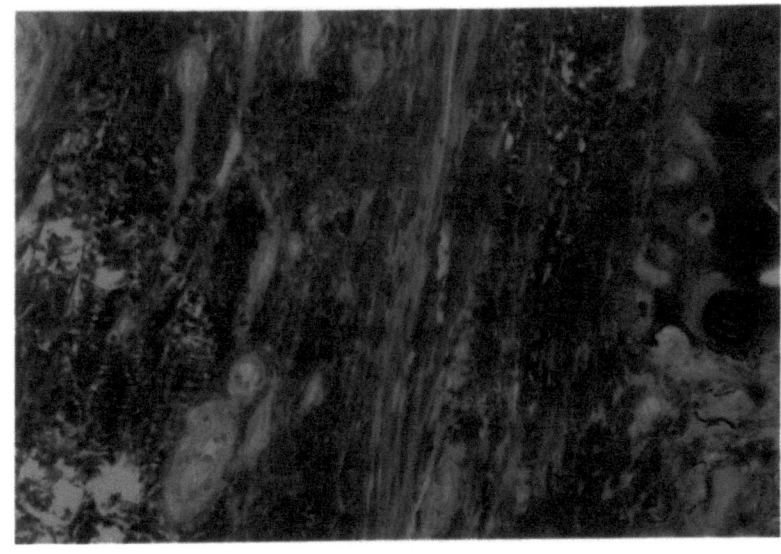

Figure 86
CC rabbit. 120 days PO. Toluidine fuscin stain. ×200 magnification (HRLM). Perivascular hyalinosis is observed, with degenerative phase of nongrafted auricular cartilage. Separation and densification of the cartilaginous intercellular limits, with abundant glycosaminoglycans, is noted.

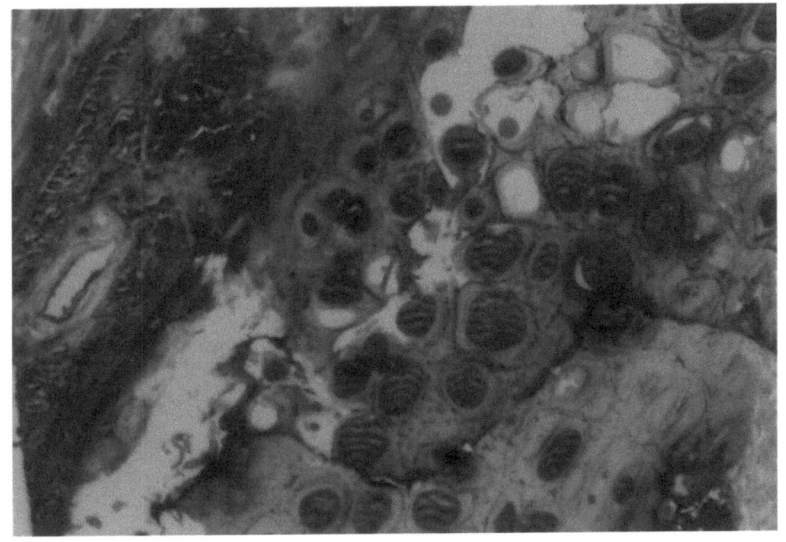

Investigation

Figure 87
CC rabbit. 120 days PO. Toluidine fuscin stain. ×200 magnification (HRLM). Necrotic areas are observed, with foci of dystrophic calcification; dystrophic fibrosis with dystrophic calcification.

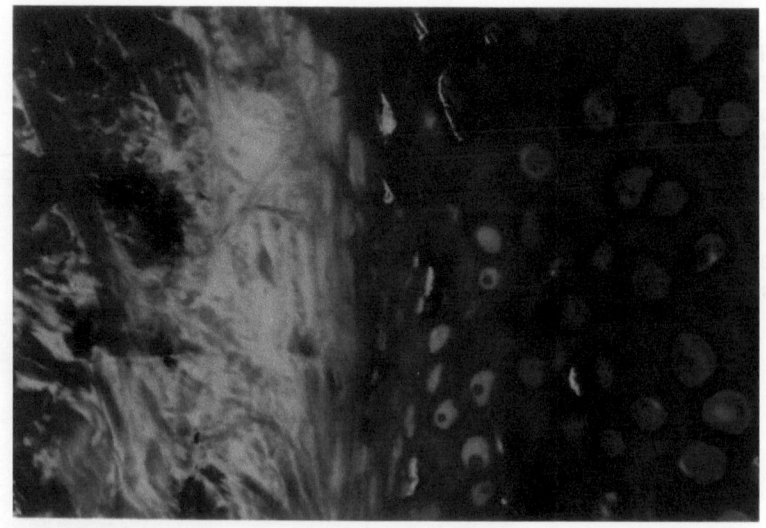

Figure 88
CC rabbit. 120 days PO. Toluidine fuscin stain. ×250 magnification (HRLM). The pseudocapsule is seen invading the chondrograft, with chondrocyte resorption from histic anoxia, and fibrous proliferation with foci of trophic calcification. Friability of the pseudocapsule is noted.

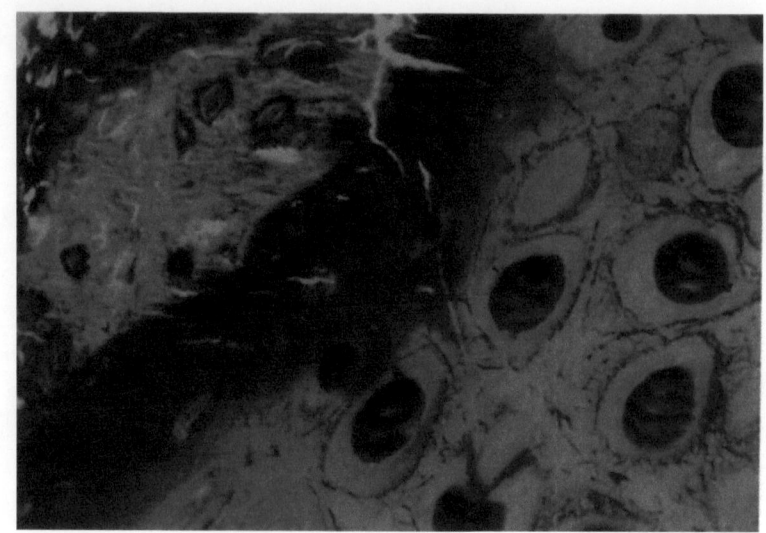

Figure 89
CC rabbit. 120 days PO. Toluidine fuscin stain. ×250 magnification (HRLM). Dystrophic edematous SMAS is observed, with muscle striation loss due to histic anoxia.

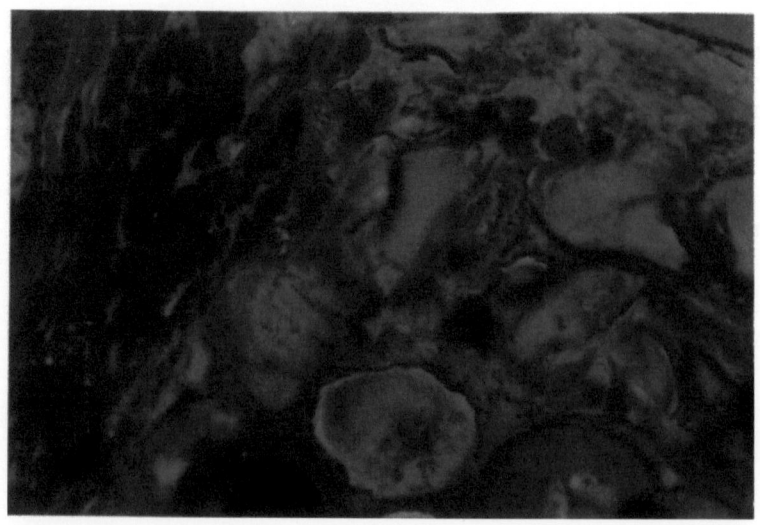

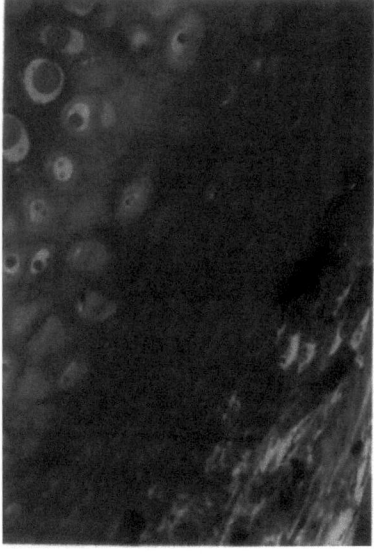

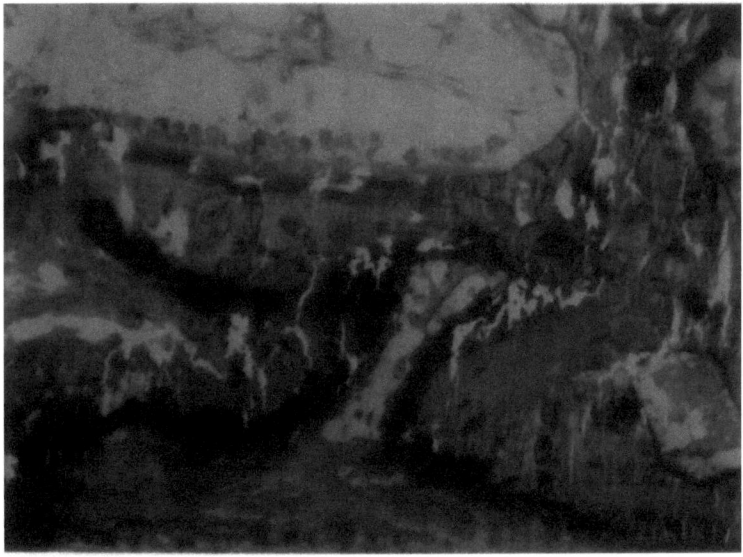

Figure 90
CC rabbit. 120 days PO. Toluidine blue fuscin stain. ×275 magnification (HRLM). The fibrous pseudocapsule is observed without trophic vessels or nerves. The muscle has atrophic and denervated fibers. There is an increase of endomicial and perimicial conjunctive tissue.

Figure 91
CC rabbit. 120 days PO. Toluidine blue fuscin stain. ×350 magnification (HRLM). Chondrocyte necrobiosis from histic anoxia. The vessel in the pseudocapsule does not reach the extracapsular limit and has intensive perivascular hyalinosis.

Figure 92
CC rabbit. 120 days PO. Osmium stain. ×400 magnification (HRLM). Axon nerve degeneration, with myelin fiber dystrophic loss. Total loss of the perivascular sheath, and abnormal proliferation of the Schwann cells, immersed in scar conjunctival tissue. Fibroblastic proliferation and deposits of primitive collagen fibers are noted.

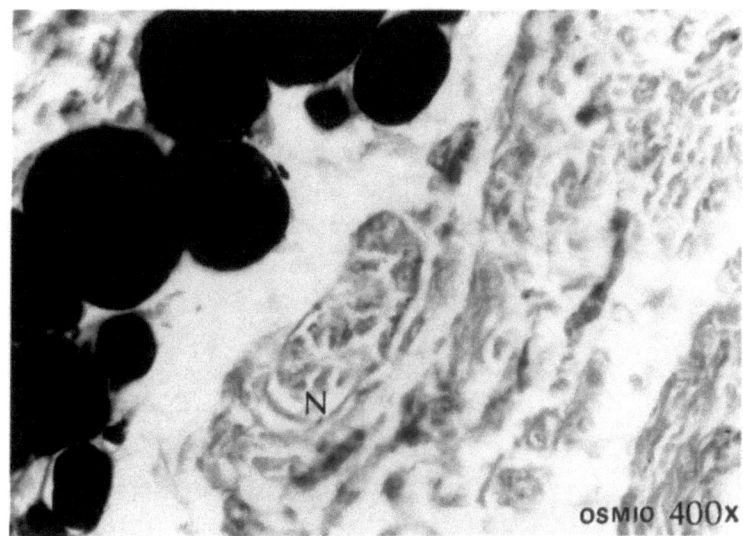

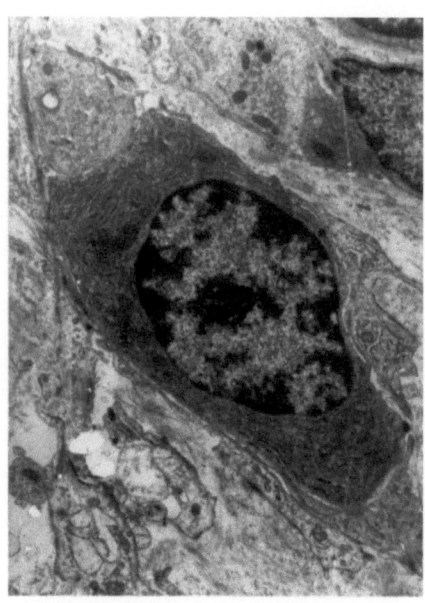

Figure 93
CC rabbit. 120 days PO. Acetate uranile-Reynolds stain. ×5000 magnification, electron microscopy. There is a relatively normal plasmocyte, with foreign body inflammatory reaction to the costal cartilage.

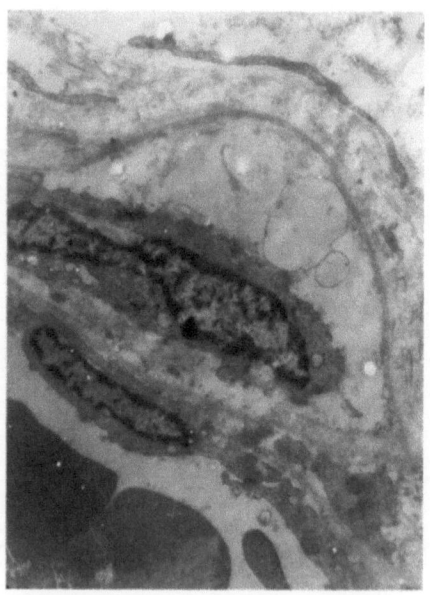

Figure 94
CC rabbit. 120 days PO. Acetate uranile-Reynolds stain. ×5000 magnification, electron microscopy. Vascular lesion, with perivascular edema, separation of the pericyte, before trophic loss (hyalinosis). Intercellular collagen fibers are noted.

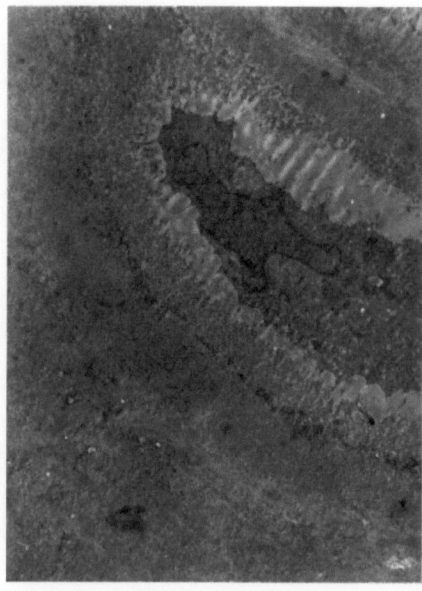

Figure 95
CC rabbit. 120 days PO. Acetate uranile-Reynolds stain. ×4000 magnification, electron microscopy. Primitive fibroblast with edema and necrosis are noted.

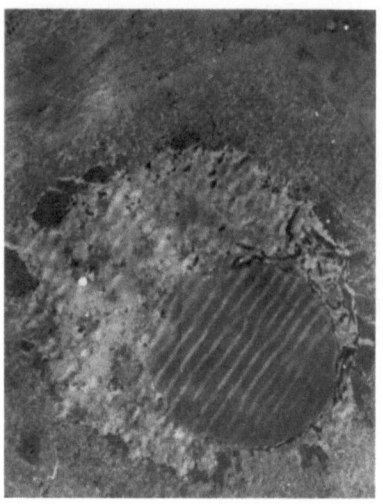

Figure 96
CC rabbit. 120 days PO. Acetate uranile-Reynolds stain. ×3500 magnification, electron microscopy. Chondrocyte with matrix necrosis, from hystic anoxia. Foci of fibrous bands are noted.

Conclusion

Findings of the foregoing investigation were in keeping with our human clinical observations, but final doubts were dispelled with electron ultramicroscopy confirmation.

In summary, grafted hyaline cartilage in the auricular area forms a pseudocapsule of fibrous tissue around the graft. Vessels and nerves do not reestablish their supply to the graft. Chondrocyte viability, both focal and grouped, was impaired with signs of cell degeneration and necrosis, areas of osteoid degeneration and calcification. Grafted elastic cartilage was observed to form a minimum pseudocapsule, perforated by vessels and nerves supplying the cartilage with neovascularization and viable nerves. Chondrocyte viability was established, including binucleation and isolated mitosis. The reestablishment of normal anatomic conditions also entailed adapted behavior of functional characteristics of the graft in the new habitat.

Once again, the laws of reconstruction have held true, establishing that an autograft is better than a foreign body, an autograft surpasses a homograft, and the best material for the autograft is the same substance.

Auricular skeletal support with silicone has faded into the glorious past, evening is setting on costal cartilage, and a new dawn has broken with the auricle made of auricular material.

Auricular Functional Properties

The habit of rubbing one's ears does not necessarily improve concentration. But from children's play to adult relationships ears have been not only something to look at, but also something to feel and tenderly caress as part of normal behavior. It is good to have them to hang your glasses on, and soft and pliable enough to lie on comfortably.

The firmness, elasticity, flexibility, delicacy, and finesse of the organ are unique, with a system of bioengineering-locked stresses due to special viscoelastic cartilage properties that contribute to retaining shape and position. The spectrum of neither auricular skin nor cartilage is duplicated elsewhere in the body. Only the skin and cartilage, muscles and nerves can reproduce auricular functions. Medical measurement of these many functions and their combinations is not easy. These functional properties are as follows:

A Sound Receptor

1. Volume: the shape cone-concentrates and amplifies sound. A special cartilage vibration is involved.
2. This volume, measured and compared on either side, gives stereo direction of sound, which is reduced in unilateral microtia.
3. With hearing education on sound direction, the patient can also learn to calculate sound distance, using the posterior bounce effect.
4. Reflex stereo by moving the head enhances this perception.
5. The concavities of the scapha, associated with the concha acting as the antechamber of the canal, contribute to sound quality: timbre, pitch, and modality.

Skeletal Formation

1. Fixation: the auricle is attached firmly to the head. The cone-shaped cartilage slides into the osteocartilaginous socket, which also has an axis curvature to hold the position. Fibrous stays are supplied by the ligaments, and further fixation is with the extrinsic auricular muscles, supplied by the facial nerve, except the deep fascicle of the auricularis anticus, which is supplied by the trigeminal nerve and related to mastication. The integument contributes as a loose container that is firmer nearer the canal.
2. Stiffness: enough to keep the auricle normally upright.
3. Flexibility: to bend and give way before a stronger force than the stiffness threshold.
4. Elasticity: the ability to return to the original shape and position.
5. Softness: supple enough to be easy to lie on.

As Organ of Sensation

1. Protopathic: perception of heat, cold, pressure, and pain.
2. Discriminative: measured by double pinpoint determination.

3. Epicritic: established by the cotton wool test. Specialized epicritic sensations (tickle, caress, erogenous) are also part of it.

An Organ of Mobility

1. Expression: the levator function is given by the auricularis superioris muscle accompanying the frontalis, and posterior auricular rotation by the upper fascicle of the auricularis posterioris contracting synergically with the risorius.
2. Sphincter: given by the intrinsic muscles, surrounding and closing the meatus. The extrinsics are antagonists and open the meatus.

A Trophic Organ: Growth, Healing

1. The sum of motion and sensation means reinnervation, and reinnervation means trophic function, because the trophic nerves grow back in with the others. The measure of trophic recovery is evident with graft growth. The upper auricle grows more during the first years of life, and the lower auricle during the later years. It is necessary to distinguish between arrested, retarded, and incomplete growth. Each has a particular cause and value.
2. The fundamental value of trophic recovery is wound healing, and is directly related to area nerve supply.

An Organ of Reflex Defense

1. Reflex to sound.
2. Reflex to sensation.
3. Combined sphincter action of the intrinsic muscles and skin.
4. The hair circle of tragus, antitragus, and Darwin's tuft contribute to enhance local reflex defense mechanisms.
5. The tragus is the guard of entry to the canal, and forms part of the meatus.
6. Cilia: movement of the hair tends to sweep the concha clean.
7. Baby suction reflex is produced when laying the ear on the mother's breast.
8. The lobule acts as a thermostat that governs body temperature through a hypophysial reflex. The lobule enlarges with age because the elderly need greater heat regulation.

Skin Function

1. Skin function is very different in the various areas. Sudoriparous glands supply moisture on both aspects, but more on the posterior. Some anterior areas, however, have very abundant sudoriparous glands and greater local sweat on approaching the meatus, and on entering the canal the glands change to ceruminous, producing wax.

2. The skin texture is full-thickness on the posterior aspect and free helical border, with normal adnexa. But it changes radically on the anterior scaphal and conchal aspects, where the skin is much thinner, more adhered, and behaves in a different way. This skin is in transition between normal surface epithelium and mucosa. It does not produce keloid, in contrast with the free helical border, posterior auricular aspect, and the lobule, which are prone to keloidal formation.
3. Along with the skin, the fat distribution and quality vary considerably. Gliding fat is found on the posterior aspect, with a fine neurovascular fascia between the two layers. This fascia is also an important trophic network. The fat is a cushion to accept pressure. The lobule has trabeculated fat, firmly padded, and excellent material to be sculpted. Fat on the anterior aspect is very scarce and directly related to the skin fixation with the underlying tissue. Fat distribution and functional characteristics become evident when the auricle swells, be it from edema or local anesthetic infiltration.
4. Particular tissue layers also make the ear subject to marked cold, progressing from paleness to freezing, congelation, and possible necrosis.

Skin Color

1. Skin pigmentation is greater on the more exposed lateral surface.
2. Color is registered with vasodilation with various hues of deep red from blushing, flushing, and inflammation to cyanosis from cold.
3. Color is pale with vasoconstriction, as with expression of anger or fear. There is a relationship between the color of the ear, chin, and tip of the nose.

Bioimmunolgic Reactions

A group of bioimmunologic reactions has been noted, including allergies, inflammation, and lymphatic drainage. They have been normally and pathologically well established.

An Organ of Delicacy

The particular touch of delicacy on both sides of the head are like other delicate formations on view, such as the nare border for the nostril, or the eyelid border. Their balance agreeably meets the eye, but the lack of balance and harmony is immediately obvious and perceived as an abnormality.

Chinese Medicine

The inverted fetus on the ear for Chinese acupuncture is a different sphere of reflex action.

A Functioning Element in Surgery

The last, but most important, of these characteristics for the reconstructive surgery is that adequate pinna reconstruction defines the best door of entry for the auricular atresia. The auricle must comply not only with shape but also with these many functional characteristics to fill the requirements of approach to the tympanic cavity.

Conclusion

These functional characteristics establish the auricle as an organ, a viscera, that is part of a system.

Pinna–Partial Canal Syndrome

I have further described a combination of upper auricular deformity associated with the subtotal blockage of the external auricular canal, and named it the pinna–partial canal (PPC) syndrome. The symptoms have been repeated often enough to establish symptomatic relationship as a syndrome. It consists of two parts. The auricular deformity affects the upper third of the organ with severe lop, severe snail shell, satyr, or canoe ears. The upper third is deficient or absent. The other part is a partial canal atresia, similar to that previously described. The canal roof is blocked by a mass of cancellous bone separated from the temporal squama by a layer of microcartilaginous fragments, muscle remains, fibrous tissue, sebaceous glands, and fatty tissue. The floor fistulae epithelium is normal for the area and filled with wax. The fistular lumen is 1 to 2 mm in diameter, and widens out deeply shaping a juxtatympanic pouch, with a normal or nearly normal tympanic membrane (Fig. 97).

Figure 97

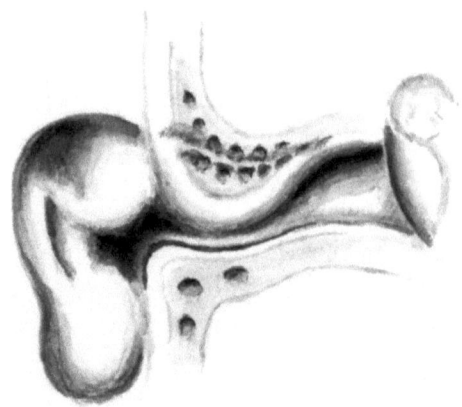

PINNA – PARTIAL CANAL SYNDROME (DAVIS)

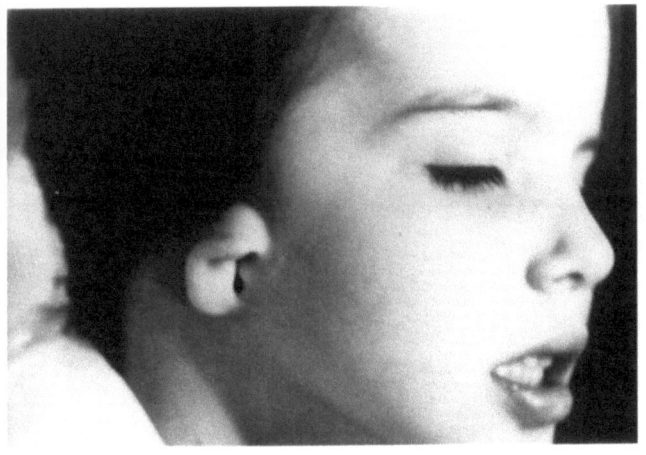
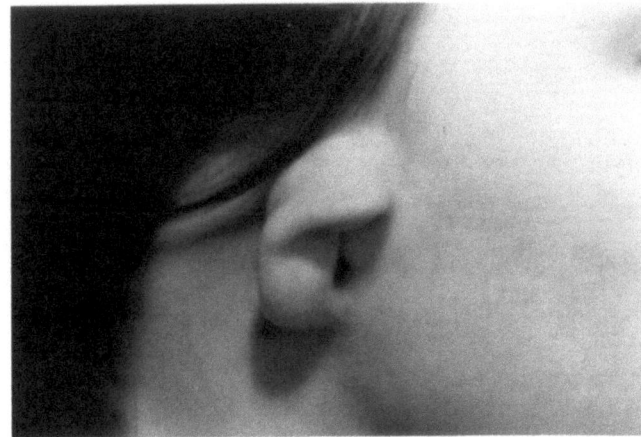

Figure 98

Case

This girl's anomaly was a severe snail shell ear with partial atresia (Fig. 98). The atresia involved a subtotal obstruction, affecting the canal roof. The floor was continuous. Her reconstruction commenced when she was 6 years of age. Her first operation consisted of opening up the shell deformity by disinserting the anterior helix and incising along the upper conchal border (Fig. 99). The upper scapha then rotated backward, and the defect became apparent. Cartilage and skin were taken from the contralateral ear, the conchal cartilage tailored to fit the defect, and was held with 6-0 silk (Fig. 100). An anterior helical cartilage strut graft was added. Surplus retroauricular skin was stored in the abdomen.

Observe how the upper skin flap was brought down over the conchal cartilage graft, so that the cartilage and skin sutures were on different levels.

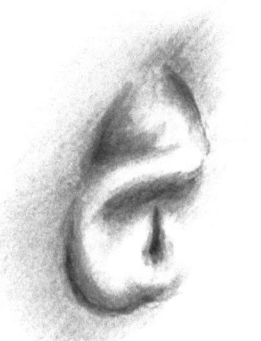

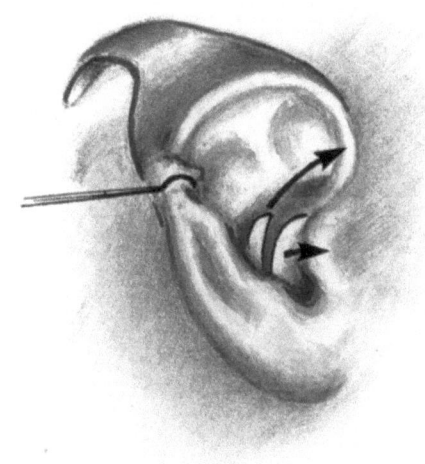
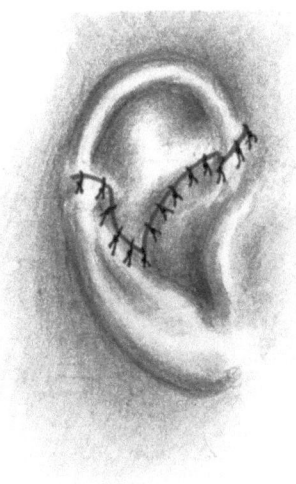

Figure 100

Figure 99

Pinna-Partial Canal Syndrome

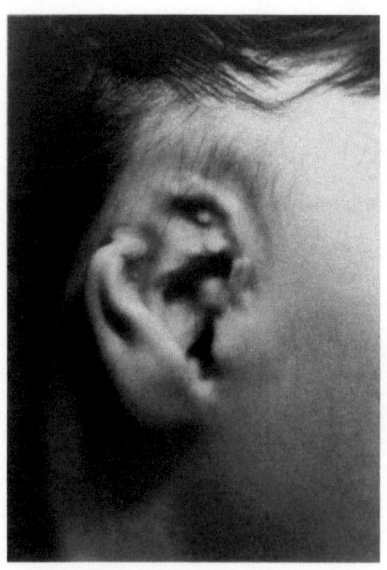

Figure 101

Figure 102

The postoperative course was good, and the result of this first stage is illustrated (Fig. 101).

At the second operation, the cartilage graft was raised, the lower helix Z-plastied, and the retroauricular skin defect grafted with ample, thick partial-thickness inguinal skin (Fig. 102).

The result of the first operation, the design of the second, and the result of this second stage are shown (Figs. 101, 102, and 104). The subtotal canal obstruction was clearly observed in the HRCT scan (Fig. 103).

A vertical incision along the canal roof provided a sufficient approach to the atresic canal, and the roof was removed with a curved gouge. The retroaural skin graft that had been stored in the abdomen was used to graft the canal roof and was held with sponges. Once the canal obstruction had been removed, a normal tympanic membrane came into view, with a juxtatympanic pouch. The postoperative course of this double operation was uneventful (Fig. 104).

At a later, third operation, some minor surgical revision was performed. Computed tomography controlled the canal caliber. Examination of the canal and tympanic membrane was satisfactory. Control audiograms are shown in Figure 105, and the patient learned to use the reconstructed ear. Hearing and audiostereognosis radically improved. Mild flexibility and retroaural sulcus depth are shown with glasses (Fig. 106). More flexibility is with moderate flexion. Maximum flexibility is demonstrated (Fig. 106).

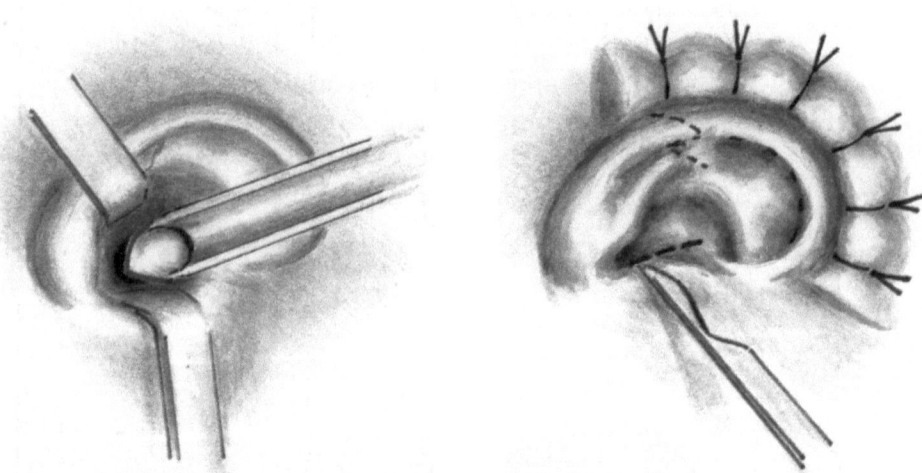

Figure 103

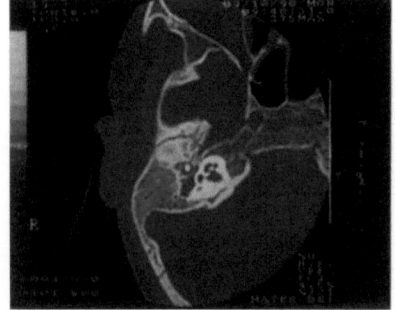
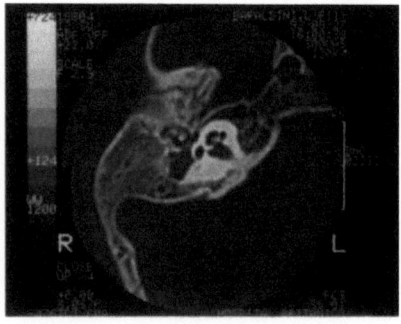
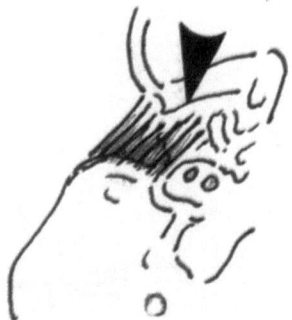

Chapter Four **The Cartilage**

Epicritic (cotton wool test) sensation was normal at 18 months and discriminative (double pinpoint test) was normal at 20 months, as compared with the other ear (Fig. 107).

The compass measures the normal ear axis (Fig. 108). The longitudinal axis of the reconstructed ear is 4 mm shorter than the normal side. This is within the measurement that Farkas has established as being unnoticed. The adequate canal caliber is shown with the introduction of the speculum (Fig. 108).

Figure 109, taken with the microscope, views the normally functioning tympanic membrane, in the depth of the neocanal.

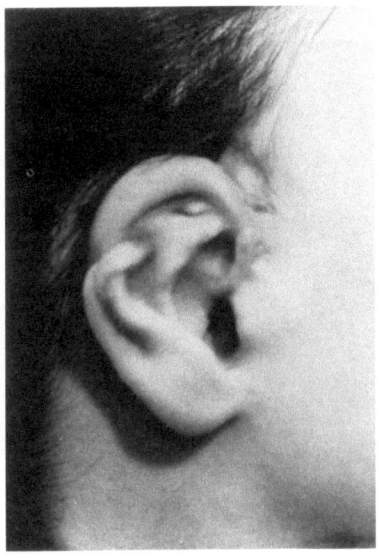

Figure 104

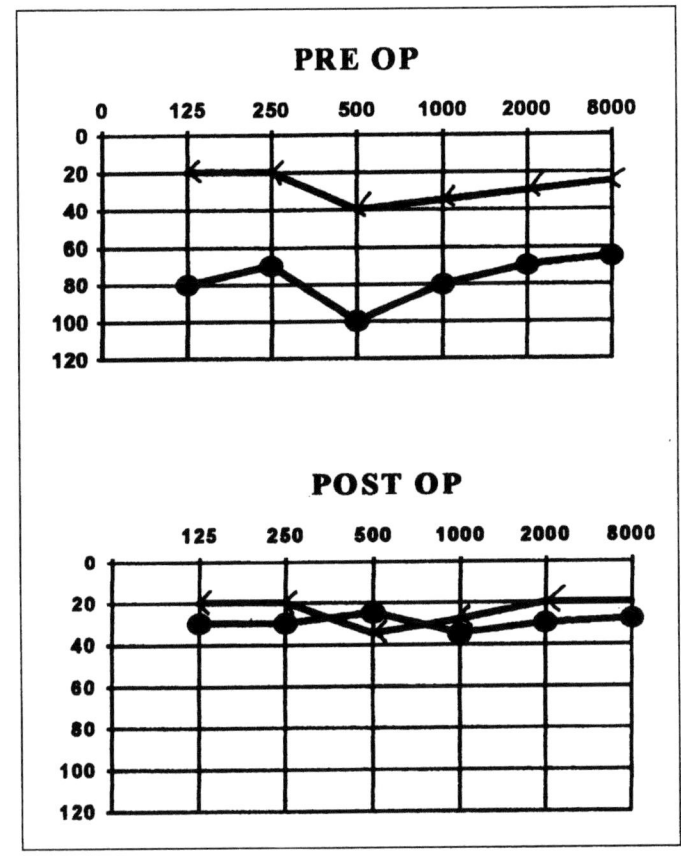

Figure 105

Figure 106

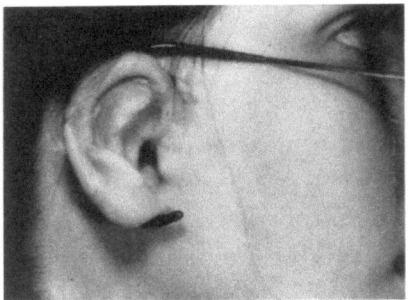
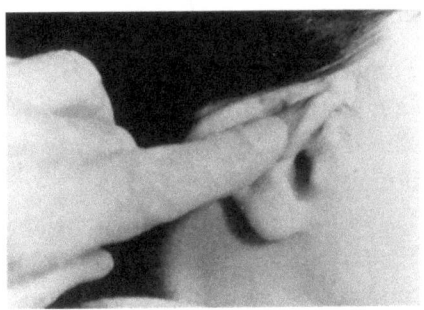
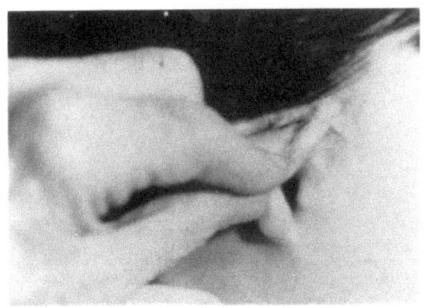

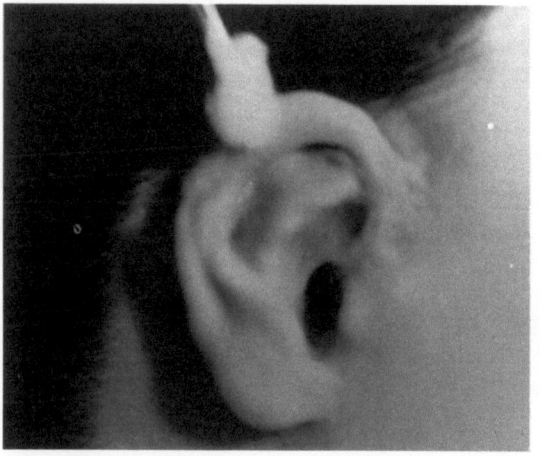

Figure 107

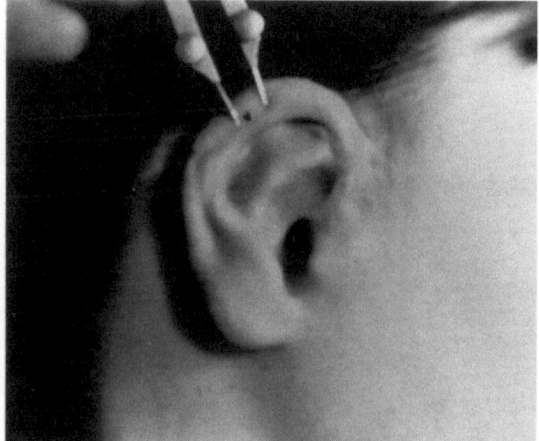

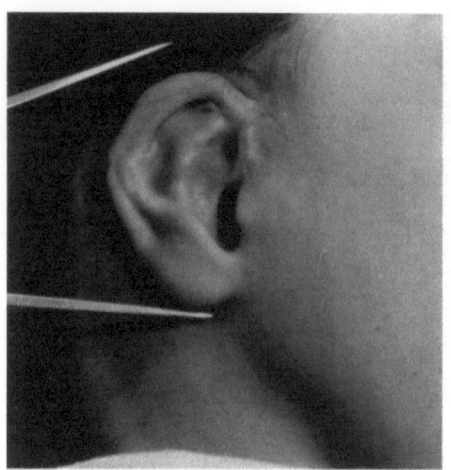

Figure 108

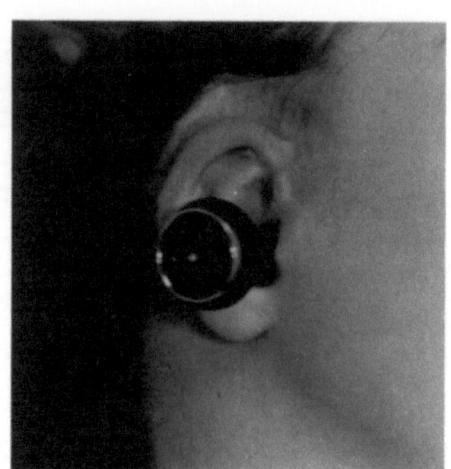

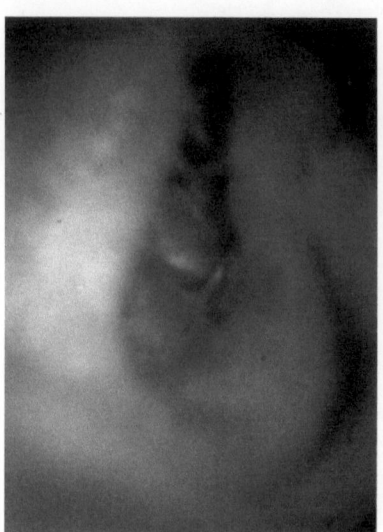

Figure 109

Figure 110

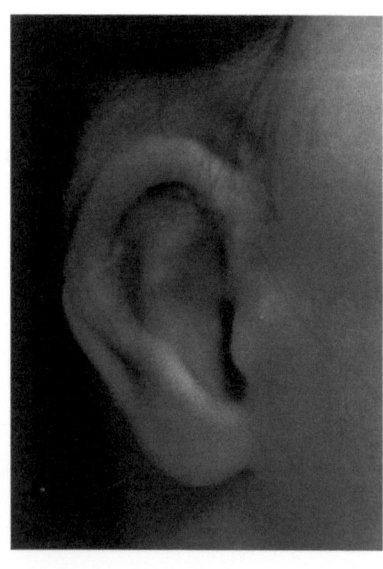

The auricular result after 2 years is shown in Figure 110. I suggested completing the repair with sideburns, but unfortunately the patient was too well satisfied with the result, and her parents preferred to decline further surgery.

Thus, the following characteristics constitute this syndrome:

1. Auricular defect in the upper third.
2. The juxtatympanic pouch is embryologically early. The tympanic ring is formed later.
3. The tragus forms part of the canal, not the auricle.
4. Preserved juxtatympanic pouch.
5. The canal floor is continuous.
6. The canal fistulae surface downward.
7. The middle ear and tympanic membrane are present and functional.
8. There are two canal segments: superficial and deep.
9. There is a relative plane of cleavage between the tympanic and squamous bone, through the synostosis.

Moderate Microtia and Total Atresia

As the scale of deformity became worse, I have chosen as an example this teenaged girl who chose a simple repair for moderate microtia and total atresia. The microtia affected the whole organ, and the lack of tragus was in keeping with the atresia. The type (canoe ear) and size of deformity are shown in (Fig. 111). But the patient did have a deep retroaural sulcus with plenty of skin, which was used to maximum advantage. The CT was favorable (Fig. 111).

Retroaural skin and conchal cartilage were removed from the normal ear, as grafts, and placed on the table.

The microtial skin was incised just within the conchal border, as designed (Fig. 113), and the upper two thirds of the microtial cartilage degloved. The intact skin bag was then turned inside out over the surgeon's fingertip, and radically defatted. With defatting the skin expanded. A long, narrow helical cartilage flap was sculpted (Fig. 112) to wrap around the cartilage graft dome, as the conchal graft was carefully cut to fit exactly and comfortably over the microtial scapha, and the cartilages were sutured together. Then the skin was draped back over the neo-framework. The helical sulcus was stretched back and up with transfixion sutures surfaced within the hairline over a bolus.

The microtial conchal cartilage was removed and grafted to shape a good-sized tragus. The maneuvers are shown in Figure 113. The contralateral skin graft was placed to expand the microtial conchal floor.

Transfixion sutures were kept in place for 25 days, until the grafts were firm, and the helical sulcus was marked. The postoperative period was uneventful.

Three months later meatomyringoplasty was performed. The canal was drilled, the atresic plate removed, and the neotympanic membrane made by grafting skin on the middle ear mucosa, right on the hamulus and lower hamulus ligament. The ossicles were functional.

A subtragal flap had been fashioned, and was brought back to cover the posterior meatal wall. The remaining raw surface was grafted with fine split-skin from the medial arm. Simultaneously, the lower microtial cartilage was tailored and set back to place the lower ear closer to the head, and reduce the prominence, by rolling it backward.

Thus, the deformity was repaired in two operations. The first involved the auriculoplasty, and the second the meatomyringoplasty. The result is il-

Figure 111

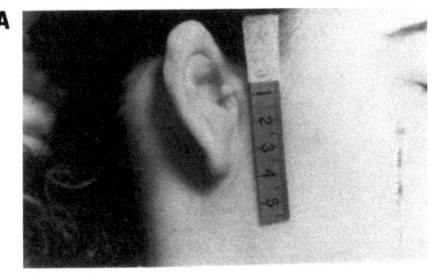
A

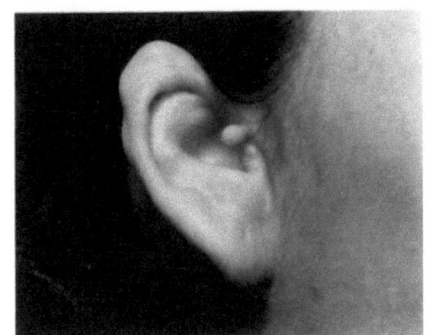
B

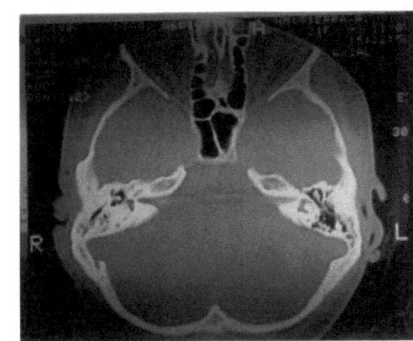
C

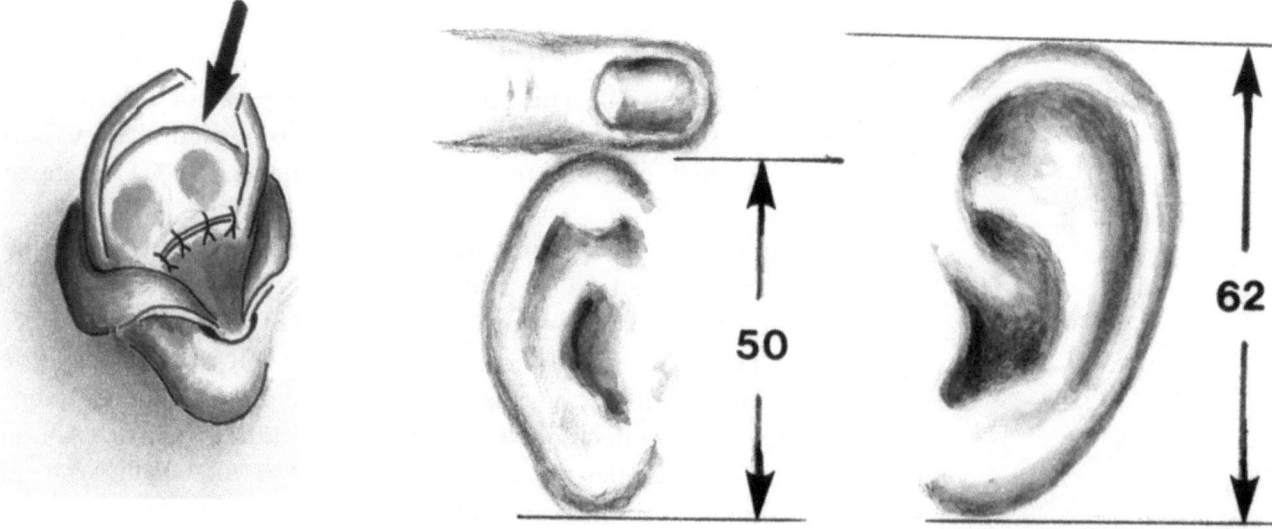

Figure 112

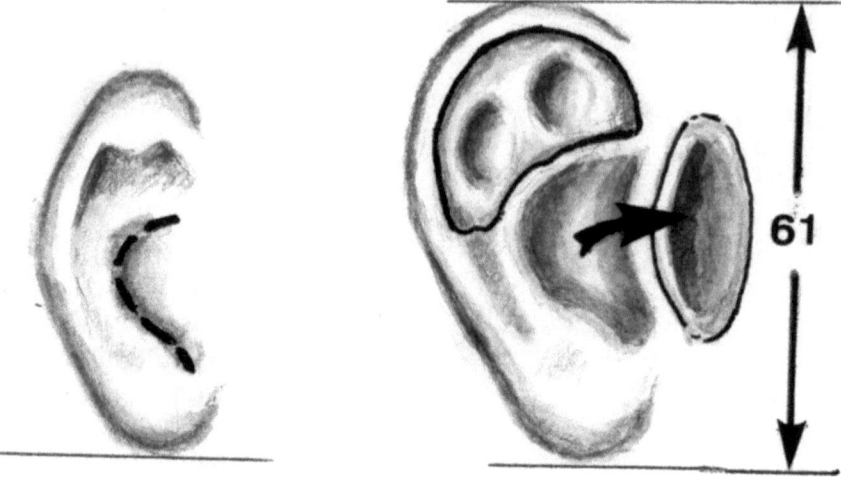

Figure 113

Figure 114

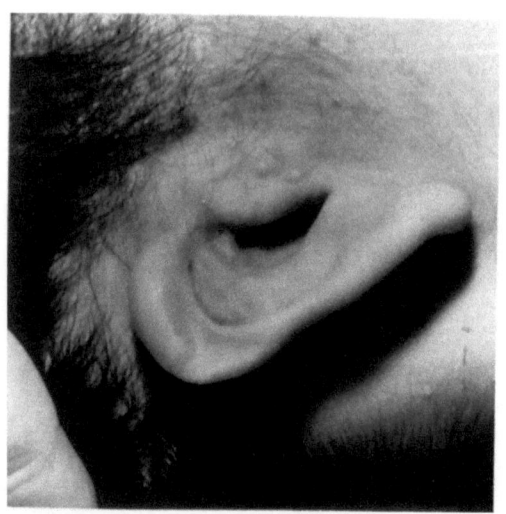
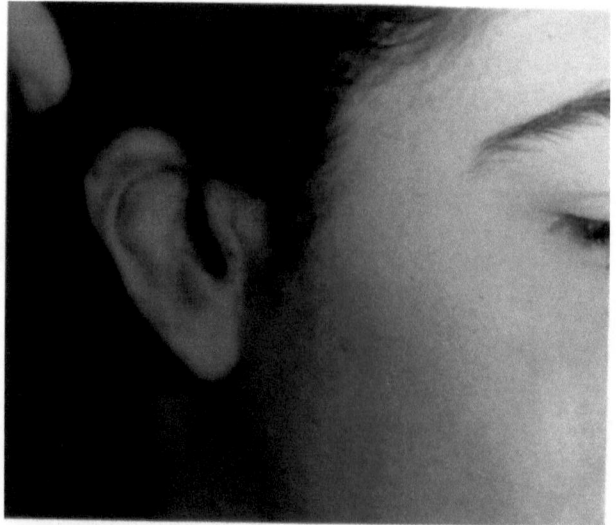

Chapter Four **The Cartilage**

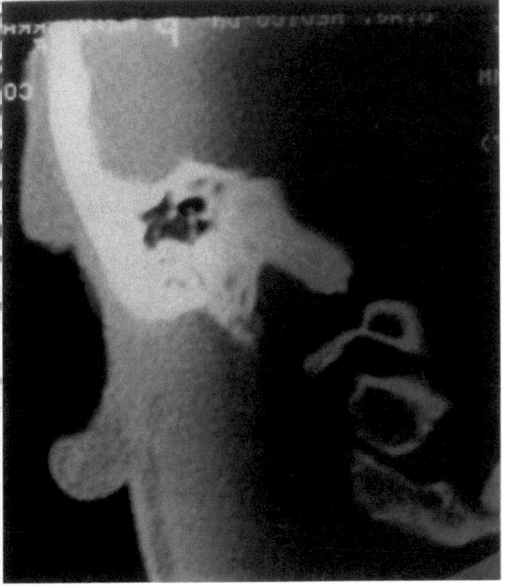

Figure 115

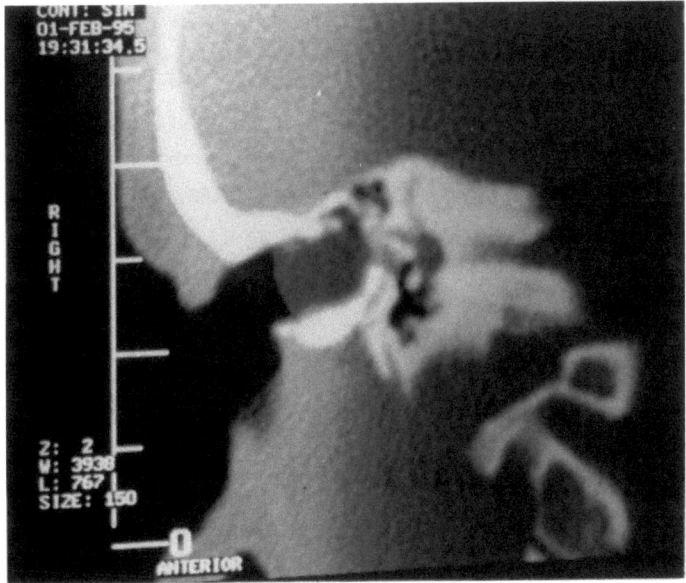

Figure 116

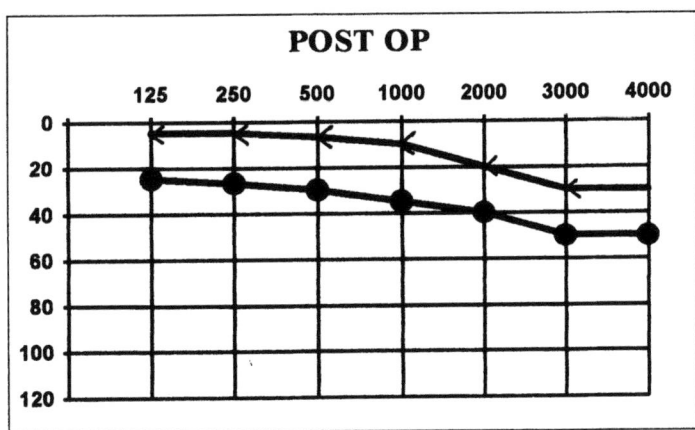

lustrated in Figure 114, with the expansion. Measurements are in millimeters. The expanded major axis had increased to 61 mm, 1 mm less than the normal side, but 11 mm more than the original measurement.

Figure 114 illustrates the result after the first and second operations. The postoperative audiogram (Fig. 116) registers the normal hearing obtained. The preoperative audiometry was in keeping with atresic conductive hearing loss (maximum 65 dB; air-bone gap at 2000). The late postoperative result (1 year) shows the gap reduced to normal levels, as graphed in Figure 116. Pre and postoperative HRCTs clearly show the canal (Fig. 115).

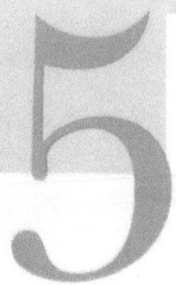

Severe Microtia and Radical Auriculoplasty

The first and second arch syndrome is misnamed. It is a first and second arch plus a tubotympanic pouch syndrome, which is a completely different matter. Unequal progress of these formations, fusing with the pneumatization at birth, reaches a working level normally after 4 years of age. Abnormally, it takes longer. Malformations of this syndrome involve three components: microtia, auricular atresia, and hemifacial microsomia. The three components are always present, to a major or minor degree, but they compose one syndrome. Diagnosis involves all three parts. Optimal treatment also includes the three parts, and entails the least amount of surgery, performed in the shortest period of time, and resulting in an appropriate improvement for the patient; it is not simply a pastime for the surgeon.

But the three parts are always one whole. Thus, the biggest problem in microtia is the skeletal support, the biggest problem in auricular atresia is the myringoplasty, and the biggest problem in hemifacial microsomia is the soft tissue repair. The mandibular asymmetry may be the most evident, but the most constant element is the parotid deficiency. The biggest challenge in this syndrome is adequately correcting the three component parts simultaneously.

Textbook anatomy is defined as the science of body structure. Microscopic magnification has added finer detail. Variants considered within normal limits have been established, and further variations constitute pathologic anatomy, detailed when embryology has burst ahead. A different conception has been introduced with the intricate study of the functions of each tissue, and surgical anatomy deals with the living organ.

Plastic surgery anatomy goes further. Aesthetic surgery is widespread today. Patchwork reconstruction may improve the monster, but it barely prepares him for normal life. Aesthetic surgery alone can suffice in simple cases, but in more pronounced deformities there can be no failure along the line of repair. In principle, it is wiser to get the right tissue to the right place, and with good substance on hand add detail and finesse. Therefore, surgical anatomy for the plastic surgeon is many things, but especially functional aesthetics. Knowledge of anthropology and social environment are also involved.

The result must justify the surgery. Plastic surgeons unversed in this subject cannot expect to achieve the necessary success, as there is no easy short cut. They should not attempt ear reconstruction, because this surgery must be correct the first time; secondary repair is bad even in the best of cases. The plastic surgeon's first step is measurement (surface measurements and deep measurements) and diagnosis. Diagnosis and surface measurements have been previously discussed by this author,* but deep measurements are especially important, gauged principally by ear computed tomography. The scanning guides diagnosis, establishing position, direction, and canal caliber for the reconstruction.

Recent developments in functional embryology and physiology of the external ear have contributed to a new outlook in otoplasty, and a new level of surgery.

Unilateral Microtia

The Donor Ear

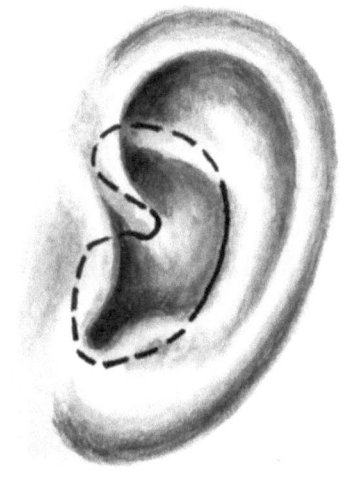

Figure 117

In contrast to the surgical technique used for conchal cartilage removal in the prominent ear, where the cartilage is unimportant but attention is focused on preserving the deep perichondrium in the lodge to reform a fibrocartilaginous conchal floor, in radical repair the conchal cartilage is all-important and removed with special care to preserve the perichondrium on both surfaces of the cartilage graft. The exact line of chondrotomy must be measured, so that the donor projection will also be used for the reconstructed ear projection. Thus, the chondrotomy incision is marked precisely halfway up the posterior conchal wall, under the lower crus and the antitragus, and anteriorly bordering the external canal meatus (Fig. 117). A blunt arrowhead is cut around the radix helicis. Half the projection remains on the rear donor conchal wall, and the other half is incorporated in the graft to contribute to the helical border projection. This is termed *precision chondrotomy* (as designed).

We have generally found that the donor ear is fairly large and prominent, and it somehow seems to be nature's desire to balance the small defective auricle. The final position has both ears fairly close to the head, for symmetry and to minimize comparison with the other side.

Chondrotomy is approached through the posteromedial auricular aspect, and the oval skin graft is removed simultaneously.

Tragus

An ample tragus is measured and marked, making maximum use of local skin adhered to the underlying cartilage. A chondrocutaneous flap is raised, but with only one layer of cartilage, to give the tragus a good shape but to keep it thin and delicate. The tragus chondrocutaneous flap thus remains in situ (Fig. 118).

---

*Davis JE. *Aesthetic and Reconstructive Otoplasty*. New York: Springer-Verlag; 1987.

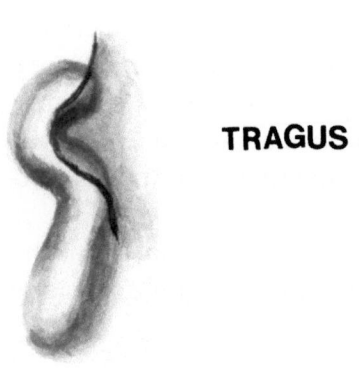

TRAGUS

Figure 118

After the microtial skin flaps has been placed, traced, and incised, calculating the approach to the middle ear, the microtial mass is reached. To accomplish this, two different skin approaches are described, one with a lobular setback Z-plasty, and the other with a continuous lobe to dome stretch of uninterrupted skin in two stages. The cartilage mass is variable, but there is always more below the surface than meets the eye. The remainder of the cartilage is then removed with the perichondrium and placed on the table alongside the contralateral conchal cartilage. Both are prepared to shape a full-sized skeletal framework, sculpting and joining them together.

The often-heard criticism that native cartilage is not enough is incorrect. In fact, there is more than enough to pick and choose the quality and quantity from the two grafts on the table. The actual assembly depends on the ability and artistry of the surgeon.

Auricular Integument

The change of epithelium in the auricular area comprises four areas:

1. Total skin, with fat and adnexa, covers the posteromedial auricular aspect, and the lobule ends at the helical border, which is the dividing line of nerve and vascular endings. For this reason, a helical border incision is practically bloodless and painless.
2. From the helical border to the external auricular canal meatus (porus) there is a transition of epithelium. This skin of transition is thin, has minimal fat, and is relatively adhered to the cartilage, with downy hair and few adnexa.
3. From the canal entrance (meatus or porus) to mid-canal, ceruminous glands abound.
4. Epithelium from the mid-canal to the tympanic membrane is a modified mucosa, without adnexa or hair, and practically without fat or desquamation.

Reproduction of the different types of epithelium covering is a necessary requirement for the reconstruction because function will thus be incorporated.

Figure 119

Covering

It is necessary to obtain the finest skin covering from the start, to mark the surface with a good final relief. After anesthetic infiltration of the scaphal area, the skin is incised as shown in Figure 119. The scaphal skin flap borders are held with hooks to aid the maneuver. A large, flat, and sharp scalpel blade is used gently to sweep exactly under the dermis, producing a skin thickness flap. The blade should go beyond the designated periphery by 5 mm, to extend the needed skin laxity. Due to this unique type of skin, and the exceptional superficial subdermal circulation of the area, the thickness is reduced radically with excellent viability. Then the flap is raised and retracted, and delicate and meticulous pinpoint microcauterization under magnification is performed for hemostasis until the wound is dry. In my ex-

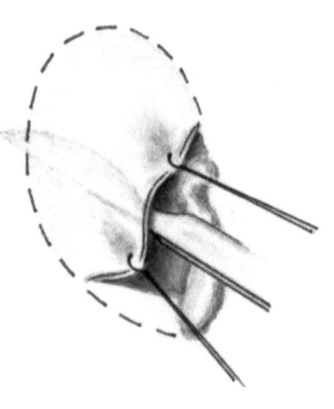

perience a sharp scalpel blade is the best instrument for uniform clean dissection, especially on reaching the hairline with changes of skin thickness. Scissors, either flat or curved, do not have the same precision, because the compression and expansion maneuvers sever irregularly with crushing blunt dieresis. Sometimes the framework anthelical axis tends to slope backward, because it follows the original radix helicis direction of the donor ear concha. This axis is reoriented by thickening the skin flap with a strip of subcutaneous tissue. It is necessary to design this strip previously on the flap, raised after framework introduction, to ensure the exact positioning of it. The strip softens the local anthelical curvature and accentuates the anthelical projection by separating the fossa triangularis from the scaphal.

With the skin flaps prepared as a covering layer, the two auricular cartilages on the table are used to construct the framework. The best type of assembly in my experience is illustrated in Figures 120 and 121. The cartilage is held border to border with 6-0 silk, and this union has stood the test of time. The rear conchal wall is raised with a sickle-shaped slice of cartilage added to the frame, which also reinforces it. Then the framework is introduced under the skin covering flaps, and tested for position, size, inclination, and symmetry.

Lobule

Customary auriculoplasty commences with retroplacing the microtic lobule as a modified Z-plasty. It is best to have abundant trabecular lobular fat in the flap, so that the earlobe is bulky and of sufficient vertical dimension to be fairly fleshy, projecting at the upper border to mark both the antitragus and contrasting depressed infratragal gutter. To sharpen the upper border, a slither of microtic cartilage retained in the flap is useful. The fat seems overabundant and bulges up, but this is just what is necessary, and it needs to be covered eventually with an extra tongue of skin from the conchal skin

Figure 120

Figure 121

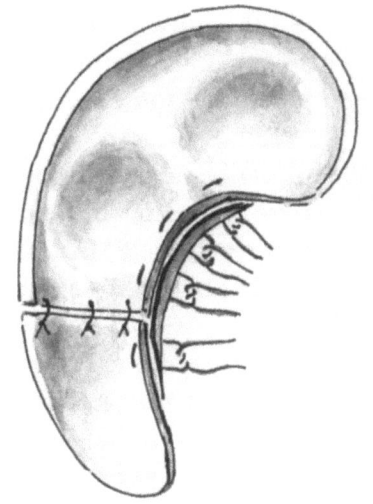
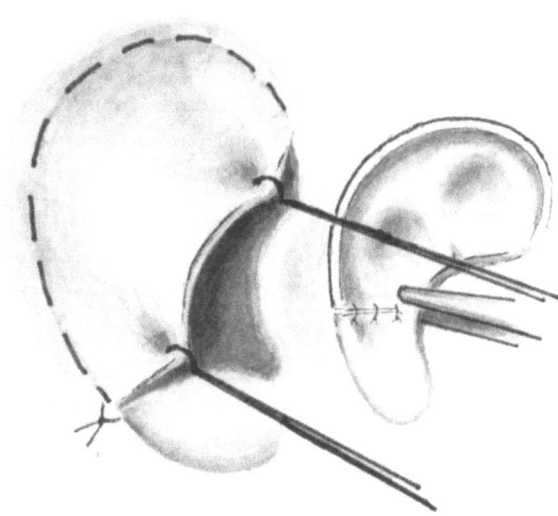

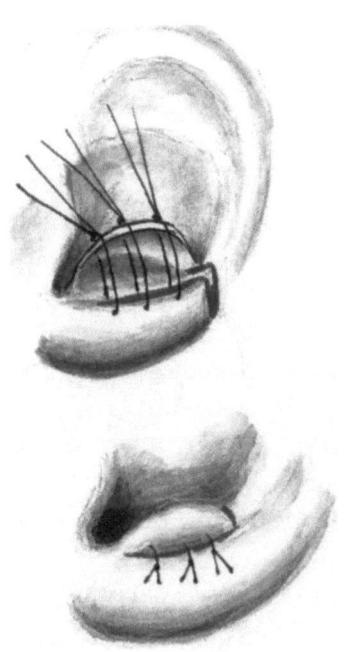

Figure 122

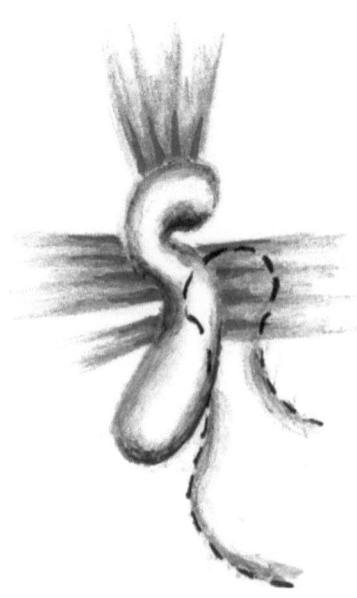

Figure 123

graft (Fig. 122). The scar simulates the antitragal gutter. The bulky fat subsides with time.

Muscle Layer

Embryologically, the original muscle formation applies the primitive traction on the shape of the cartilage mass. Two strands are strong, the eventual auricularis anticus and superioris. They drag the cartilage open and the antechamber of the canal results. The concha is probably further opened later with mastication. On deepening the antechamber to form the concha, the posterior border has been bent by gentler traction to form the anthelix. The auricularis posterioris is weaker and divided into two fasciculi, so that the posterior border is only curved, in contrast to the anterior section, which is sharply flexed to form the lower crus. The position of the canal meatus has also contributed to this difference.

The auricle should be defined as a viscera, belonging to an apparatus, and therefore should comply with definite functions. Every viscera is supplied with a membranous adventitia that carries the visceral vessels for survival. In the case of the auricle the adventitia is the SMAS, with the superficial temporal, auricular posterior, and occipital arteries. The superficial temporal supplies the tragus and external auricular canal floor, reaching the tympanic bone and spans over the lateral part of the canal. It thus divides the external auricular canal into two segments: the lateral of epidermal origin and the deeper of modified mesoderm.

Another fascia supplies the concha via the posterior auricular artery, derived from the second branchial arch. Both fascias join at the tragus border. These fascias later develop the intrinsic muscular system, with the function of defining the bioarchitectural lines of tension and strain that shape the cartilaginous reinforcements of the viscera. SMAS movement is given by the extrinsics, as shown in Figure 123.

Considering that the anatomy dealt with by the plastic surgeon is alive and functional, with careful observation during surgery a fatty layer is found immediately surrounding the cartilaginous mass, but below this fatty layer a muscle layer routinely overlays the mastoid fascia. The center of this muscle layer is over the temporomandibular joint, and the muscle fibers radiate from there forward, up, and backward. This layer corresponds to the union of the auricularis anticus, superioris, and posterioris muscles, as part of the area SMAS.

Below this SMAS, occasional muscle fibers have been seen bridging from the mastoid insertion of the sternocleidomastoid muscle to the temporalis quite close to the periostium; isolated fibers reach the SMAS layer, and there are considerable chondromuscular insertions between the crumpled cartilage and the SMAS.

The SMAS, however, is surgically defined and should be used for reproducing function. Sensation and mobility that have been obtained in the neo-organ also carry trophic fibers along with them. Flushing and paling are added to facial expression. The trophism has made that viscera part of the patient. It gives the patient life with added expression. The auricle becomes more than something slapped on the side of the head when function becomes apparent.

Reinnervation

Muscular movement entails reinnervation. Recovery of sensation entails reinnervation. Normal reinnervation means trophic normalization, chiefly measured by growth and healing potential. Normal healing potential opens the door for simultaneous auricle, canal, and neotympanic membrane reconstruction.

Davis Tests

Auricular Movement

Anatomically, the frontalis muscle continues laterally with the auricularis, with a small but variable space between them. They combine in elevation function, with parallel fibers. Both are supplied by the facial nerve. Normally, it is remarkable to observe that on forcibly raising the eyebrows, the auricles go up, too (Fig. 124). This test has been applied in practice, in keeping with the concept of functional auriculoplasty.

The value of this test in surgery is to diagnose and define the myoplasty of reconstruction. It is especially useful in measuring the progress of neuromuscular recovery. In aesthetic surgery it plays a part in enhancing expression.

Figure 124

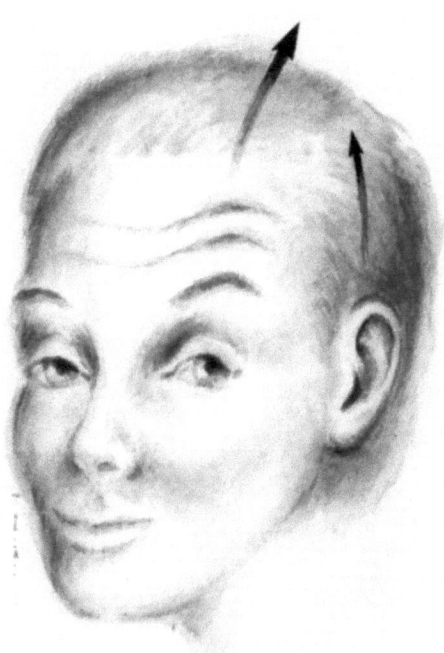

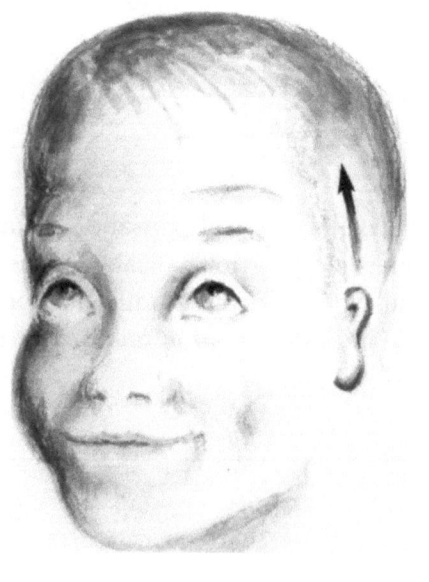

Figure 125

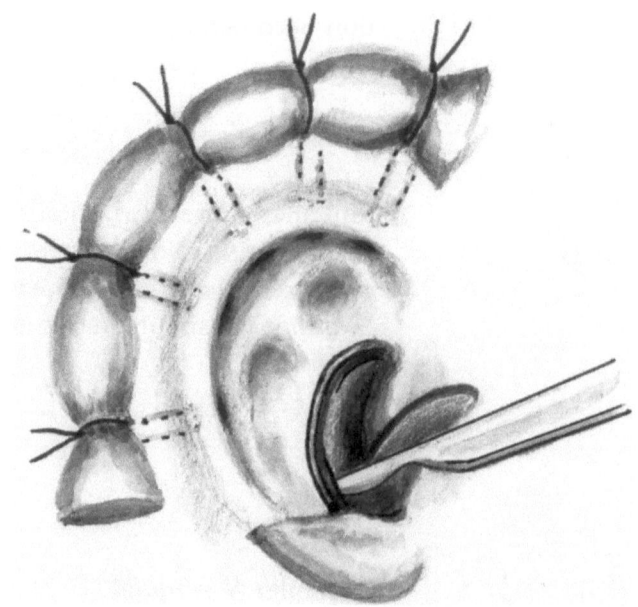

Figure 126

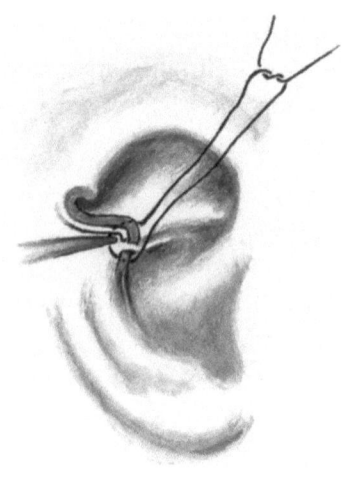

Figure 127

Microtia

When a child with microtia looks upward and forcibly raises the eyebrows, the microtia moves up, too (Fig. 125). The synchronic contracture of both frontalis and auricularis superioris is registered, and it becomes an index for local SMAS repair, for determining where and how much muscle should be included in the auricular reconstruction.

Treatment of SMAS to incorporate movement into the auricular reconstruction is obtained by preserving the remaining muscle after removal of the central area with the conchal scoop-out, and suturing the muscle stumps to the cartilaginous graft border.

The SMAS excision and myoplasty technique are illustrated in Figures 126 and 127. The sutures perforate the skin flap and chondrograft above, biting through a good portion of muscle and then piercing the conchal skin graft below.

When final healing has taken place, the action of these muscles produces some normal movement of the reconstructed auricle, both elevation with contraction of the auricularis superioris, and posterior rotation due to the auricularis posterioris. Chondro-SMAS repair contributes to revascularization, in keeping with trophic nerve supply that goes along with the new vessels.

Helical Sulcus

To shape, deepen, and maintain the helical sulcus, the following details should be kept in mind.

1. At the first operation the helical flap is uniformly and evenly reduced to skin thickness, neither more nor less. The dissection

should surpass the designated auricular periphery, extending about 5 mm beyond it.
2. After pinpoint hemostasis, three or four transfixion stitches, each a strand of 4-0 braided nylon thread applied with a long needle at each end, are used. The needles pierce the skin flap completely at about mid-scapha, pass through the cartilaginous graft border, and surface again well within the hairline, to be tied lightly over a sponge bolus. It is preferable to tie the knot only at the end of the operation (Fig. 128).

The sutures draw the scaphal skin flap in, up, and back, plicating it to form a crease, creating the helical sulcus.

Surgical Sequence

At the first operation after the conchal scoop-out, the mastoid periosteum remains visible behind and above the temporomandibular joint. The area of osteotomy is marked and the periosteum incised and retracted toward the temporomandibular joint, so that the bone surface remains bare. The cortical bone is then removed with chisel and gouge sized to fit the case. The bone is removed in one piece to be used as a graft.

The bone graft is sculpted to fit into the temporomandibular mastoid surface, by detaching and raising the area periosteum, and placing the bone graft into the slot as shown (Fig. 129).

Figure 128

Figure 129

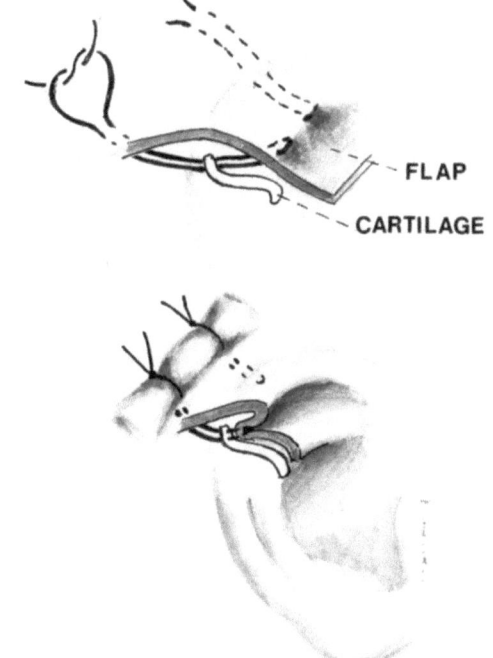
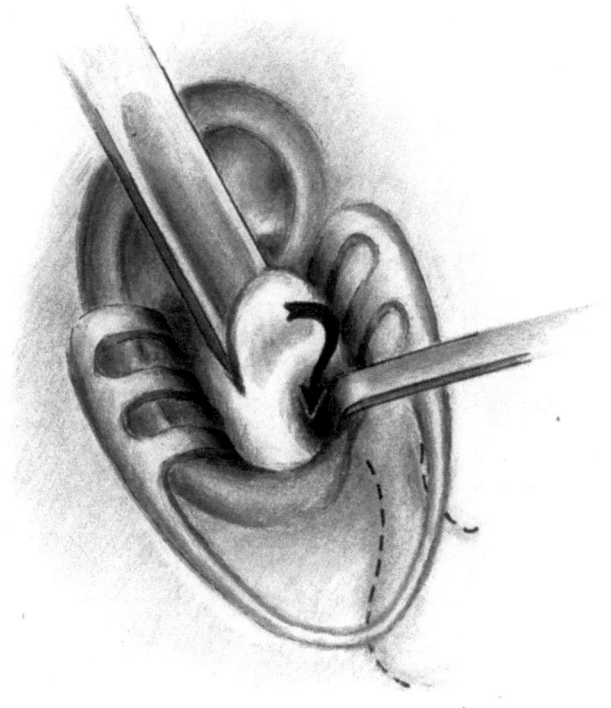

In this way, the second operation is prepared at the first operation but predefined before going in the second time.

At the second operation, performed about 4 months after the first, and when healing is well established and swelling has subsided, four factors are addressed:

1. The *postauricular sulcus* is radically deepened and covered with a skin graft. I prefer to remove a fairly thick split-thickness graft taken from the inguinal area. The advantage of an inguinal wound is that it can be closed in layers, with continuous 4-0 monofilament nylon sutures that go from one end of the wound to the other, and surface, biting deeply into the wound borders layer by layer. Four layers of running sutures are best, bringing the skin edges together so they can finally be gently joined with 6-0 silk. These running sutures are removed easily and without discomfort after 15 to 20 days. It is advisable to have the patient keep the waist flexed to relax tension on the inguinal wound borders, for 15 days postoperation. Thus, the inguinal donor site is repaired without any permanent suture or foreign body remaining in the wound.

2. The *helical sulcus* tends to flatten and become erased, so it should be deepened again at the second operation. To do this, the free helical border is incised and the flap again dissected to the sulcus. The dissection again raises a full-thickness skin flap, and all excess tissue between the flap and the cartilage is removed. The helical border is rolled back in to create the sulcus again, and is held with the same thread on two needles, passed through the sulcus depth, biting the cartilaginous border, and skin graft (covering the retroaural area). The thread is knotted loosely, but the strands are kept long to be used for the skin graft "tie-on" dressing (Fig. 130). The second deepening of the sulcus usually proves to be permanent. In the early postoperative period the helix is swollen, but when it subsides the final result is good.

Figure 130

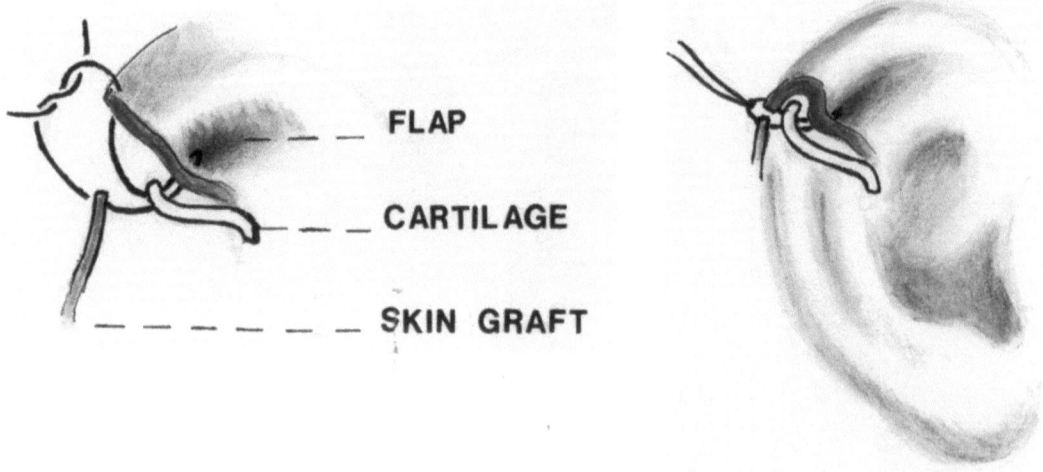

3. The lower postauricular defect is covered by radically advancing a fine *cervical flap* as a "face lift." The flap should reach right up behind the lobule to the postauricular middle third, so that eventually no skin graft remains visible and normal skin is seen. The result has been excellent.
4. Then the *canal* is addressed. The microscope is brought in, with the otologic team on hand.

It is now generally accepted that this syndrome repair should commence with the auricle reconstruction. But that immediately gives the plastic surgeon the responsibility of ascertaining detailed information about how and when and where the otosurgeon will operate. He must know what will be coming next. Both surgeons should consider hemifacial microsomia correction. There is no such thing as isolated or independent specialization. Each surgeon must interlock with the other; only then is there teamwork, step by step. The plastic surgeon must be knowledgeable about tympanoplasty and myringoplasty in order to work with the otosurgeon. The plastic surgeon must also have detailed knowledge of anatomy and pathology of the middle ear, and must know the results of computed tomography (CT) and hearing tests. At the first operation, he must place the auricle appropriately for the future canal construction. He must know exactly how much space is necessary and exactly where the otosurgeon will drill; thus, they both study the CT scan together to define the approach. The plastic surgeon must cover the canal site with a good-sized tragus. He must work with the otosurgeon to form a skin cover for the canal.

On preparing the second stage, sufficient time should elapse between the two operations for swelling to subside, so that definitive shaping of the auricle can be performed. The type of swelling and progress of the healing process is specific to each patient, and the *healing potential* varies. The conchal skin graft will thus be adequately delayed to survive as a skin thickness flap of the finest texture for the canal. A minimum of 3 months is advisable between these two operations.

At the second stage attention must be paid to the facial nerve. We now think that there is not one but several facial nerves with different functions and anatomic positioning; they are not merely branches of the original trunk. These facial nerves vary greatly, and care must be taken to avoid damaging them. Neuroexcitation is fundamental, and neurostimulators should investigate contractures continually throughout the surgery.

Preoperative CT scanning must be carefully analyzed before, and again during surgery for maximum drilling information. This means meticulous step by step burring. The scanning alone, however, is only used to localize the nerve in its neuriduct or ducts. Otosurgeons have observed the facial nerve or its branches loose and bridging in the tympanic cavity, covered only by the mucosa. Branches have been found to emerge close to the mastoid surface. They are especially difficult to work with when compacted into the limited space of the eburnated middle ear. The variety of findings need careful exploration by the surgeon not to spare the use the stimulator.

The microtia described in Figures 131 to 135 has been reconstructed with the method previously outlined, in two stages. Skeletal supports were

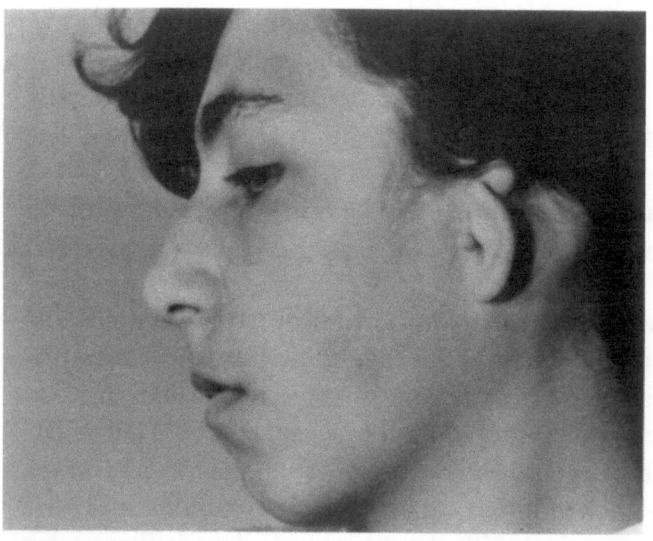
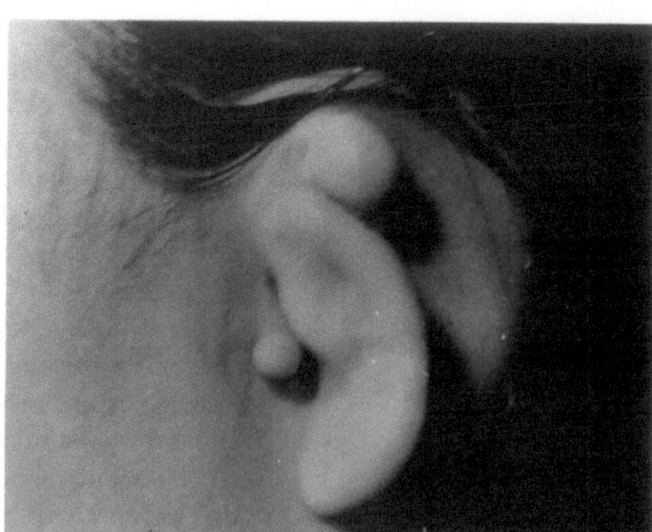

Figure 131
(Patient referred for surgery by Dr. Horacio García Igarza.)

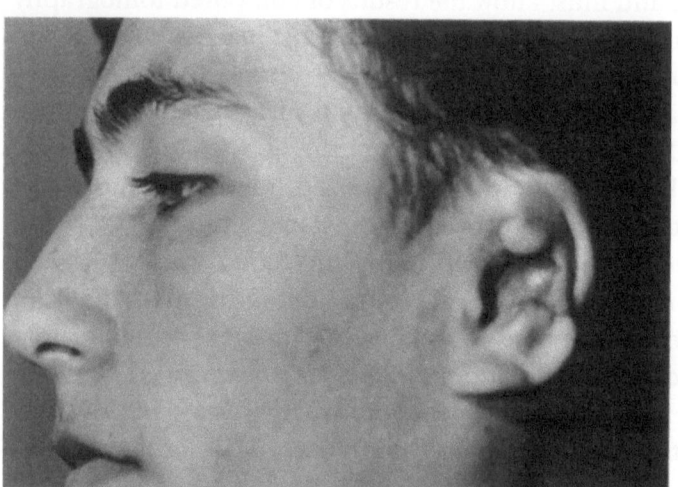
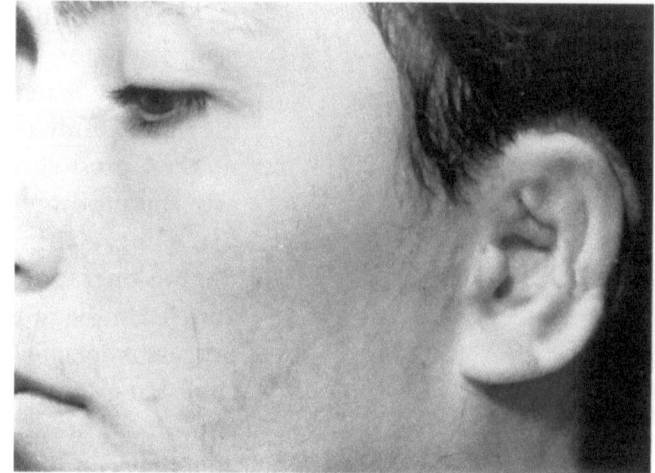

Figure 132

Figure 133

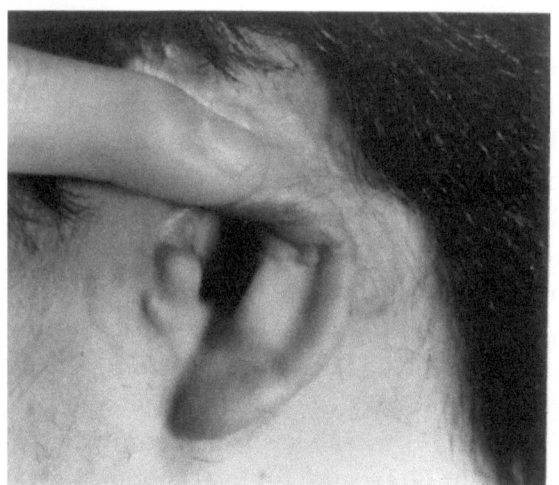
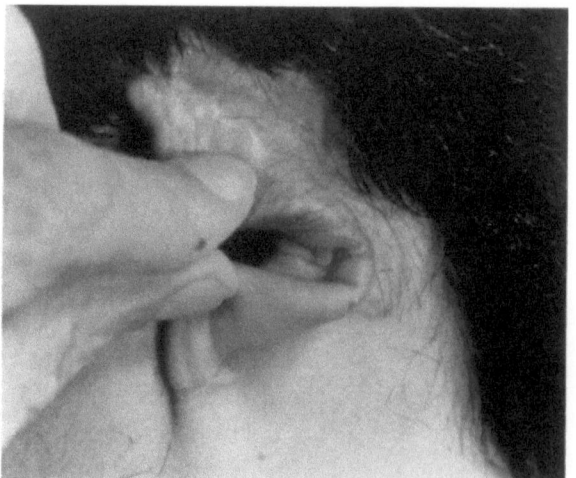

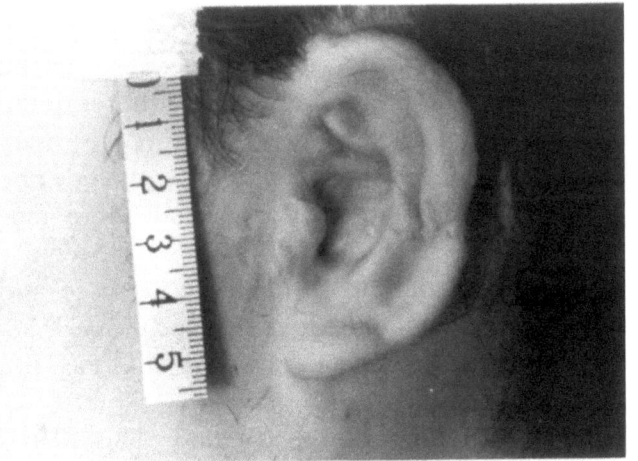
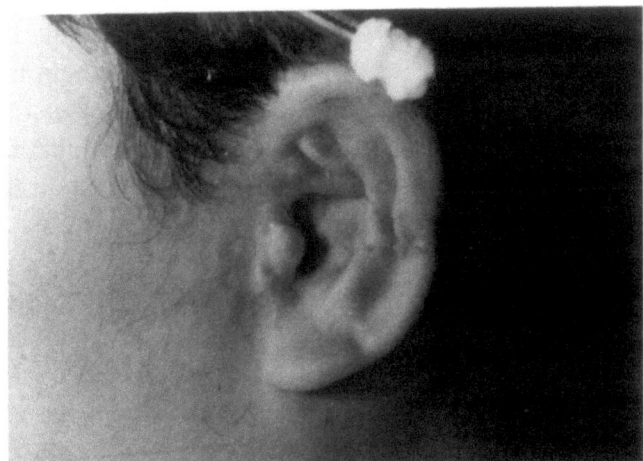

Figure 134

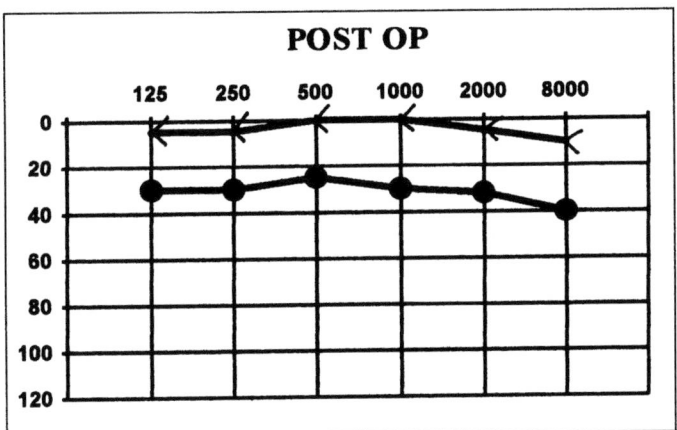

Figure 135

done with contralateral conchal cartilage, SMAS was incorporated, and the concha was grafted with retroaural skin from the normal side. Auricular elevation has been by deepening the retroaural sulcus with a fairly thick inguinal intermediate skin graft. The stage results have been photografted, and the basic functional characteristics illustrated. At a third stage meatomyringoplasty was performed, with satisfactory results.

The method described in this case left an evident scar between the lobe and scapha. This is a very common surgical sequela. The scar is visible because the texture and thickness of the skin is different on each side of it. The step deformity cannot be prevented. But to avoid this scar I have devised methods to keep an uninterrupted sweep of skin from lobe to dome, as a two-stage lobular construction.

The best of these methods is the "neolobe sandwich" method. By degloving the microtial lobular fat, scooping it out, and brining it down pedicled at the lower insertion with excellent blood supply from the inferior auricular vessels, it has provided the necessary lobular bulk. A conchal skin flap is shaped with a lower pedicle so it can be brought down to wrap around the fat flap and line the neolobe. Both flaps are held in position deeply in the skin pocket, with fine percutaneous transfixion sutures tied very lightly

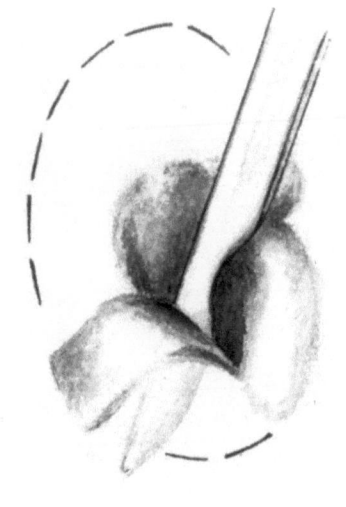
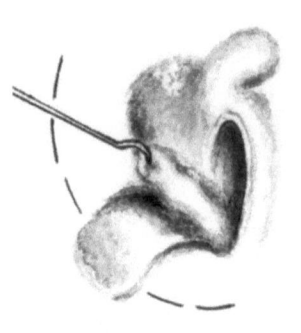
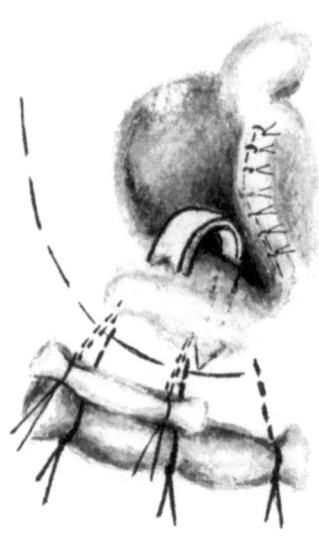

Figure 136

over sponges when faced downward, as shown in Figure 136. The finesse of the lobular shape is in the carving.

The remaining lobular microtial skin is well used to construct the tragus. Because of the special trabecular fat formation that adheres to the skin, the lobular flaps can be well sculpted and provide the necessary saliency for the tragus. A good intertragal notch is thus accentuated. The posterior conchal skin edge is then dissected as discussed above (see Covering).

At a second stage, the lower border of the lobule is released and shaped. The conchal fundus is closed so that the lobe remains properly adhered to the cheek, and the cheek scar itself raised with a mild face lift, which becomes part of the second stage.

The following case shows the result of this method. This 6-year-old patient had a "peanut" microtia and total atresia. The lobule had been repaired by the double-flap two-stage method; observe that there is no scar dividing the scapha and the lobe. The framework was made with contralateral conchal and microtial cartilage, as described previously.

The preoperative condition (Fig. 137) is shown at 6 years of age, before the three-stage surgery was performed, including auricle and canal. Figure 137 then shows the patient at 9 years of age, and at age 16. The value of this procedure is the good long-term result.

The *flexibility* acquired is controlled with eyeglasses and partial and maximum ear pligation. Figure 138 shows how the ear will yield enough comfortably to support the eyeglasses, and the flexibility and elasticity is demonstrated by bending the ear progressively. The degree of flexibility is categorized as mild when the ear comfortably supports eyeglass earpieces, moderate when the dome can bend down to touch the mid-ear, and maximum when the dome easily touches the lobule.

Sensation is examined for epicritic (cotton wool test) and discriminative (double pinpoint expansion test), and both were normal 2 years after surgery (Fig. 139). Tickle and caress sensation normalized a little later (Fig. 140).

Elevation of the ear was measured by the compass, demonstrating the muscular action of the auricularis superioris (Fig. 141). Normal growth is shown by the measurement compared with the size and growth of the other ear (Fig. 141). Both ears had grown symmetrically, as demonstrated by the open compass arms spanned to compare with the major axis of the normal contralateral auricle. The transillumination demonstrates the delicacy of the tissues (Fig. 142). CT scan control shows the neotympanum, which was functional (Fig. 142). Below it, the middle ear has adequate ossicular formation.

Audiometry improved 30 dB (Fig. 143), and audiostereognosis was normal. The patient led a full and normal life (Fig. 143).

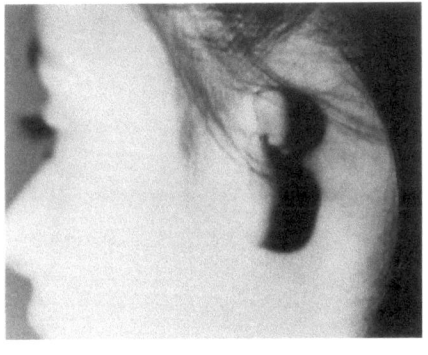 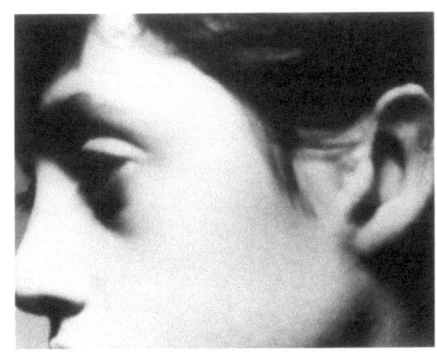 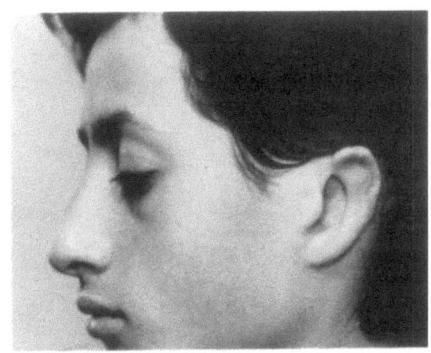

Figure 137

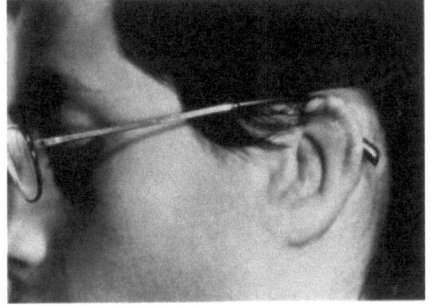 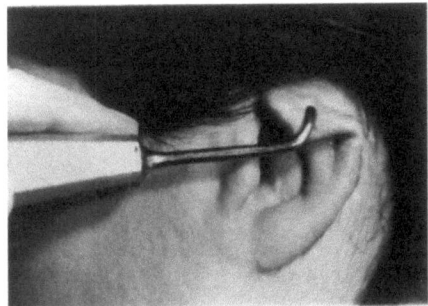 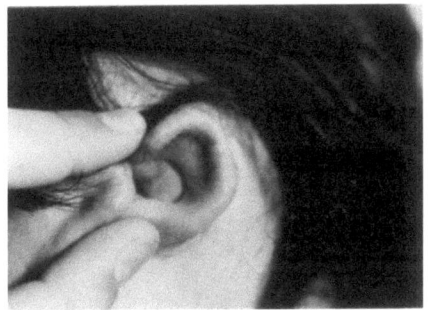

Figure 138

Figure 139

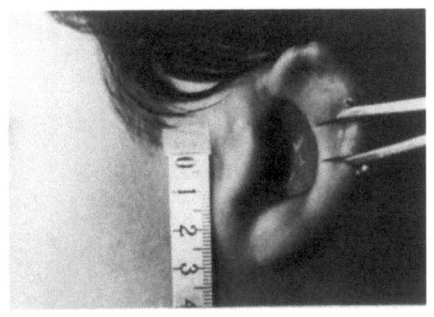 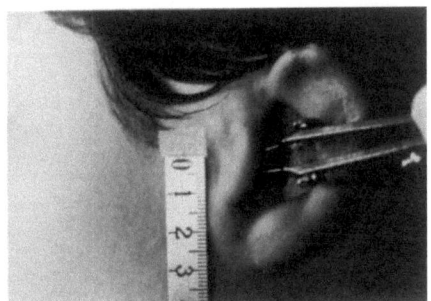 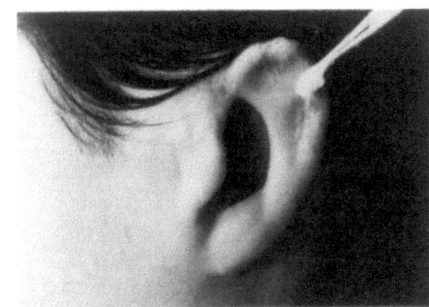

Figure 140

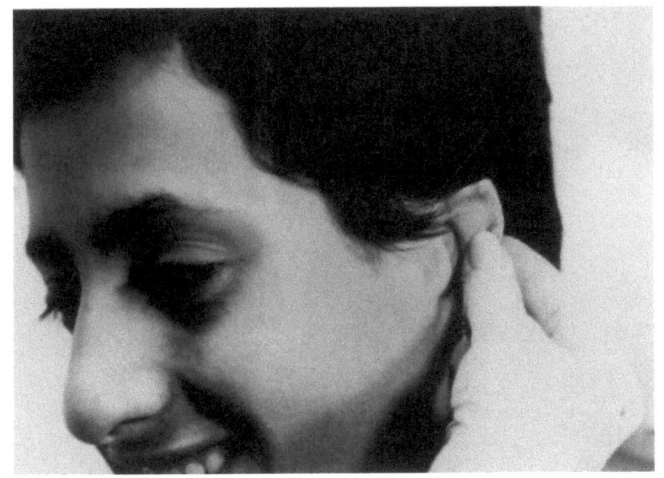 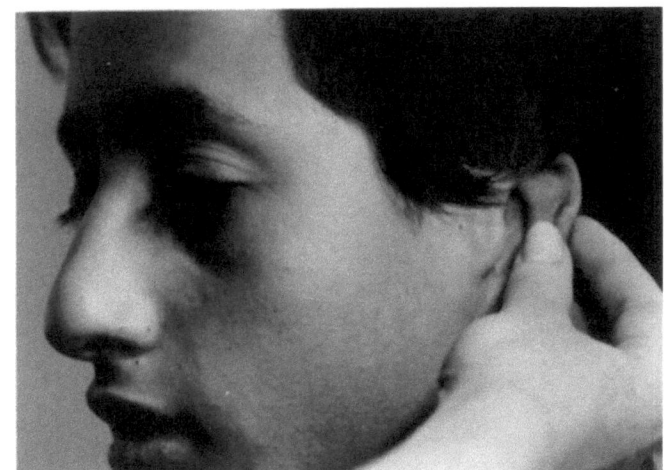

Helical Sulcus

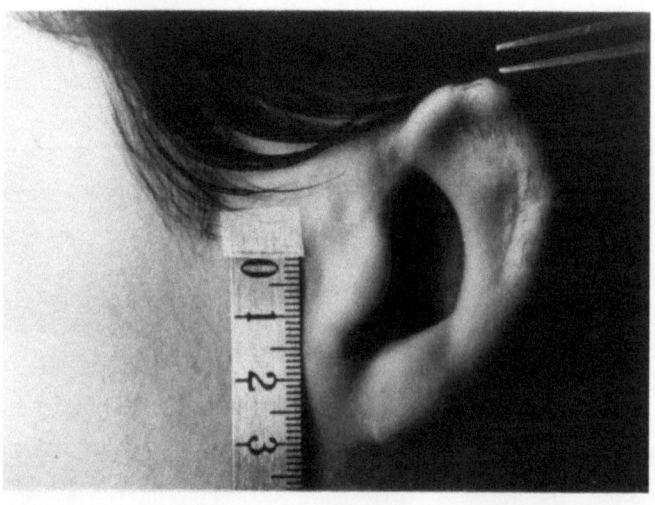
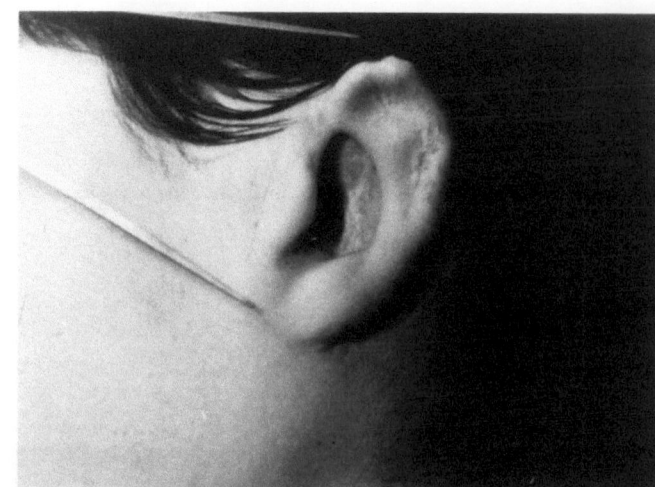

Figure 141

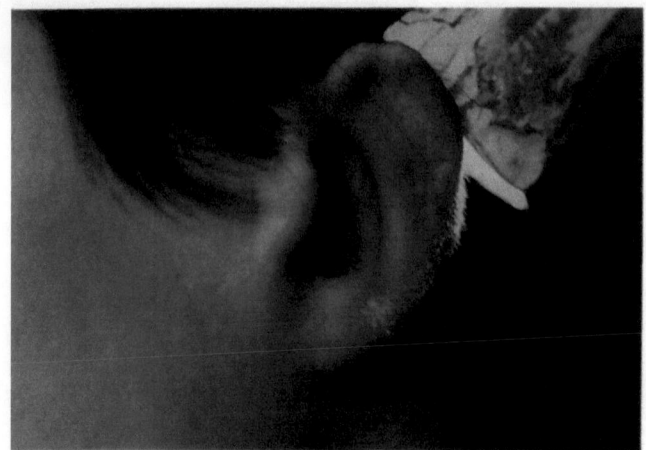
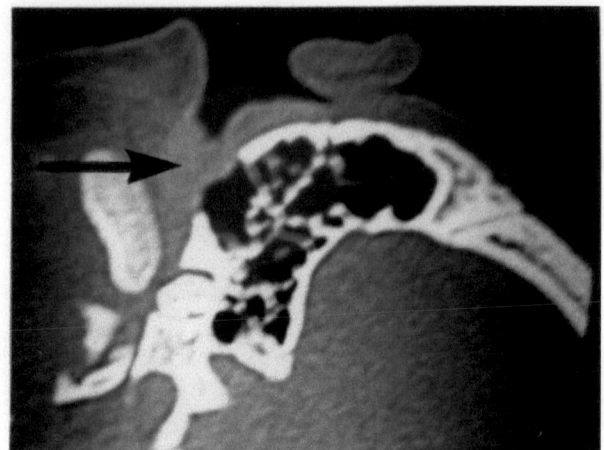

Figure 142

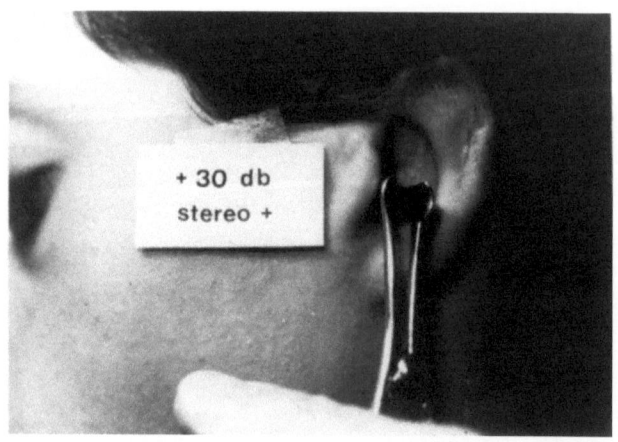
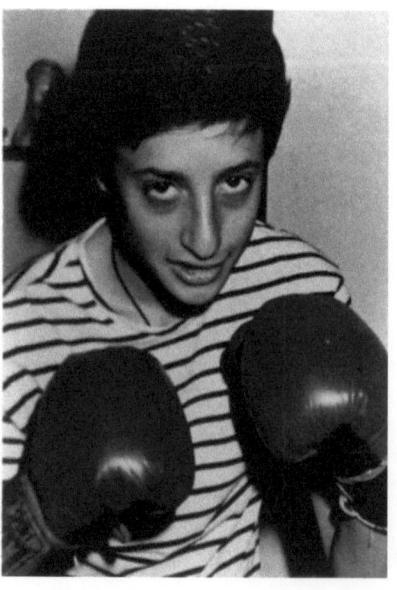

Figure 143

Chapter Five **Severe Microtia and Radical Auriculoplasty**

Figure 144

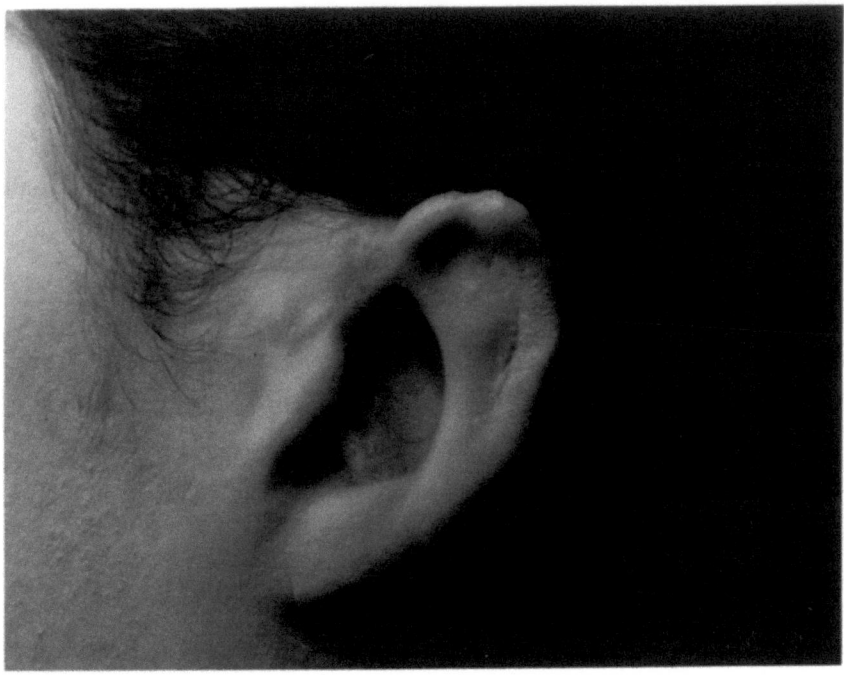

Result

Figure 144 demonstrates the ear's appearance 10 years after reconstruction.

Growth

The following sequence illustrates chondro-graft growth. The microtic patient has been photographed after birth, six months after auricular reconstruction with the method previously described, at seven years of age (Fig. 145), and then again later at fourteen and twenty-one years of age (Fig. 146). Growth of the reconstructed ear axis was measured, and increased 7 mm, during that time. It was always symmetrical with the normal ear. This observation of growth has been the rule with auricular chondrograft.

Figure 145

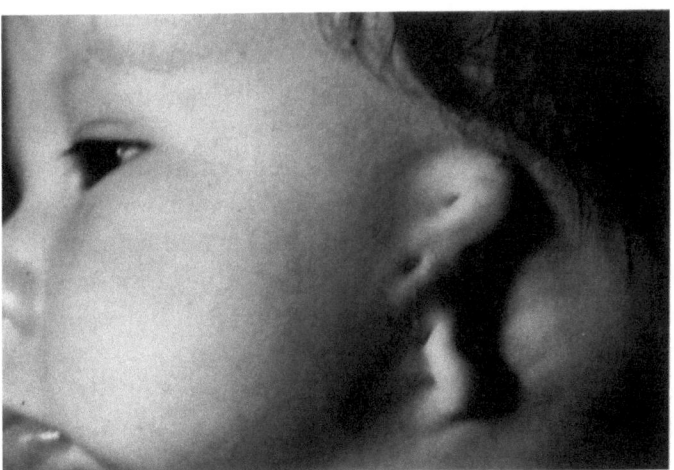
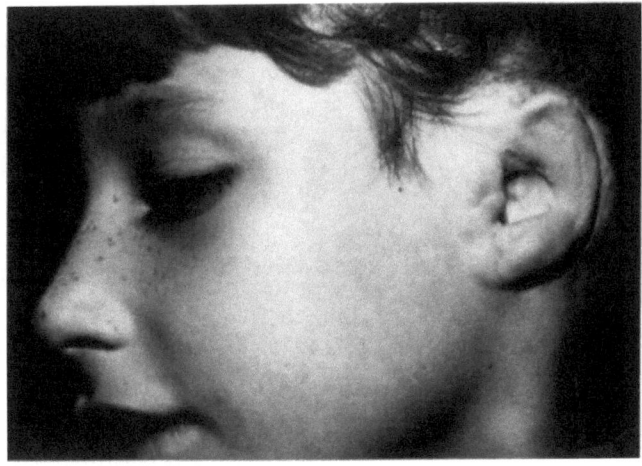

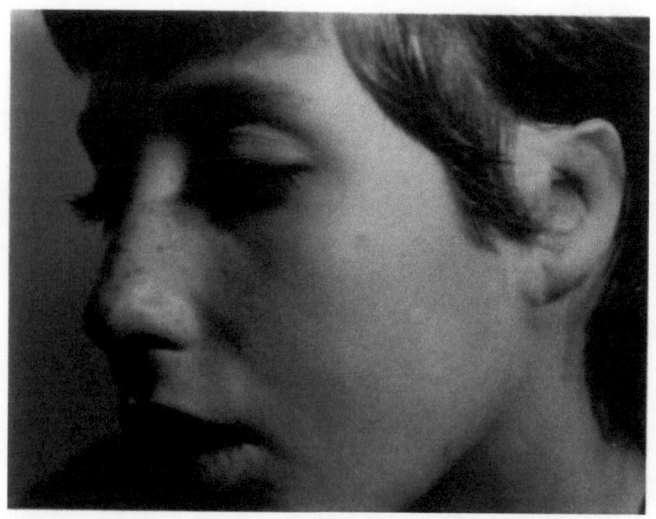

Figure 146

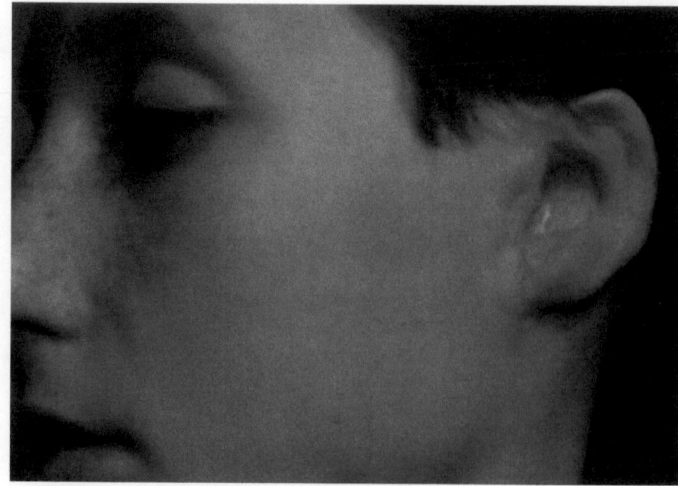

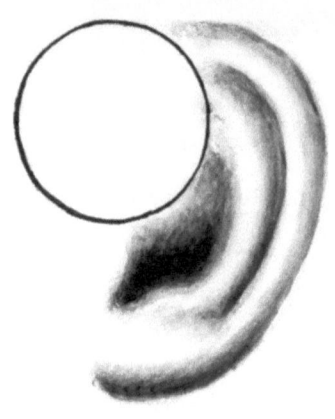

Figure 147

Figure 148

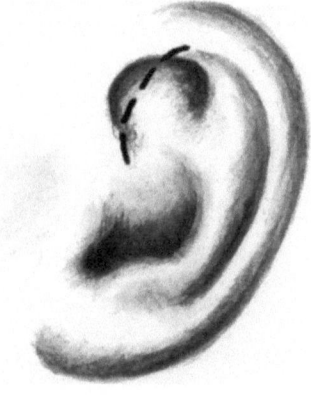

Apart from the aesthetic importance, there is a deeper value. Growth is a sign of trophic recovery. This comes from the trophic nerve fibres growing back in with the other nerves and capillaries. It is part of reinnervation.

Late Revision

A group of cases, ours and those of others, with common deficiencies, have been controlled. They usually involved a lack of definition of the anterior helical sulcus, poorly marked anterior helix and radix helicis, and an inadequate lower crus.

Figure 147 shows the defective area with a circle, and Figures 148 to 151 illustrate the surgical methods that have been used with satisfactory results in this and other areas.

The use of the upper nubbin sometimes can be included as a third stage, or with the canal construction. But usually it is a late consideration.

The balance of the depth of the helical sulcus is also usually a late evaluation, after edema has subsided. A SMAS roll can be effective either as a primary or secondary maneuver to pronounce the concha.

In some cases, the upper microtial node is fairly fleshy and full. At the first operation, once the cartilage had been removed, a sack of very beautiful skin with a considerable amount of underlying subdermal fat remained. The node was kept this way, occupying the fossa triangularis with some "memory" of shape. No further dissection was carried out so that the upper auricular blood supply was preserved. The scaphal color was so good that it was practically normal, notwithstanding the helical and conchal maneuvers of the initial surgery. At the second operation the node was not touched, and only the retroaural skin graft was incorporated to deepen the postaural sulcus and raise the auricle.

The third and final operation was for definitive finesse of the area. Figures 148 to 151 show the approach through an incision corresponding to the future anterior helical sulcus; the node was radically defatted and

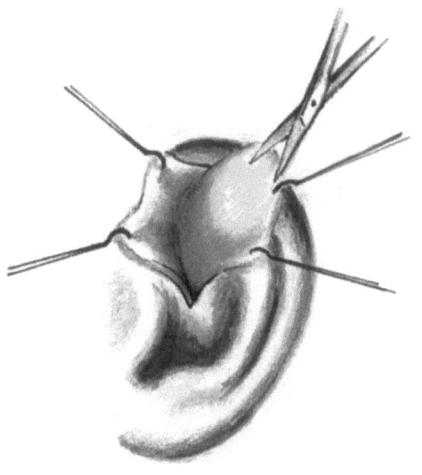

Figure 149

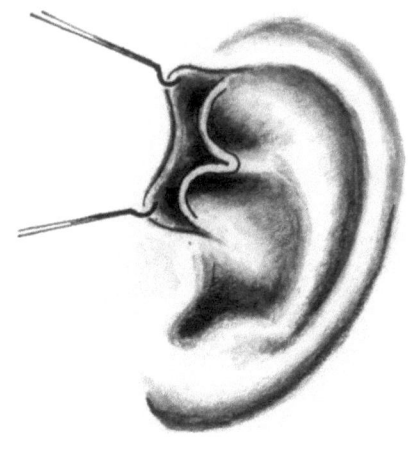

Figure 150

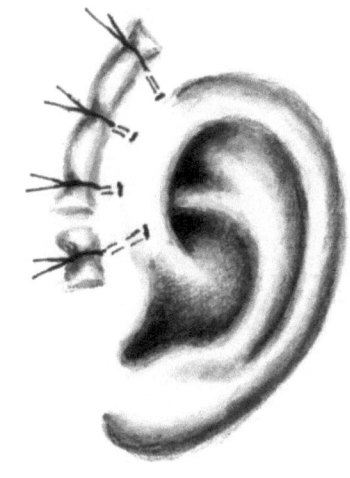

Figure 151

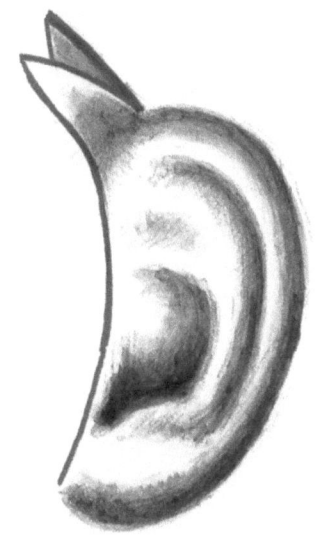

Figure 152

Figure 153

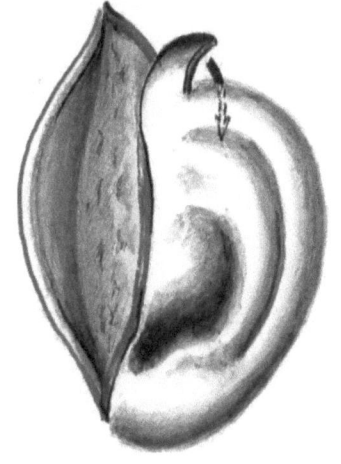

shaped to form the fossa triangularis and the anthelix. On raising the anterior wound border the skin was turned in and inverted into the helical sulcus. The node flap was advanced under it into the helical sulcus. Both fell well into place and were held with transfixion sutures tied over a bolus. A slight excess of the node flap was tailored at the lower border and turned down to form the radix helicis and the cymbal fossa, and held by a single independent bolus transfixion suture. These finishing touches completed the necessary details, but without changing the tragus.

When the tragus is also deficient, the following method has been used successfully. Figures 152 to 155 illustrate the stages of repair. First, a triangular hairless flap before and above the dome is raised, reduced to skin thickness, and a "lifting" flap, connected with the previous one, is dissected preauricularly. The first flap is turned down and into the deepened anterior postaural sulcus, to cover it. This flap holds the auricular dome slightly away from the head and supports eyeglass earpieces comfortably. The lifting flap is raised, advanced, and inrolled around the tragus to give it substance and shape.

Upper and lower tragus limits are undercut to anchor these two points to hold the lifting flap in place, and they are held with two sutures. The surplus flap above and below these points is then tailored to delimit the anterior helix and arrowhead the radix helicis, as seen in the figures. The excess flap below the tragus is simply prelobularly removed as a triangle.

The two anchor sutures mark the anterior auricular sulcus and the intertragal notch, and the remaining wound borders are sutured with the finest silk.

The importance of the anterior auricle (anterior helix, triangular fossa, radix helicis, tragus, and meatus) is that it provides the most pronounced relief and therefore throws the deepest shadows that detail the organ. But the borders that mark this relief are variable. For example, the lower crus curls down but the radix curls up around the cymbal fossa. The lower crus hangs and normally tends to drape down, but the radix helicis has to be sustained to keep its shape.

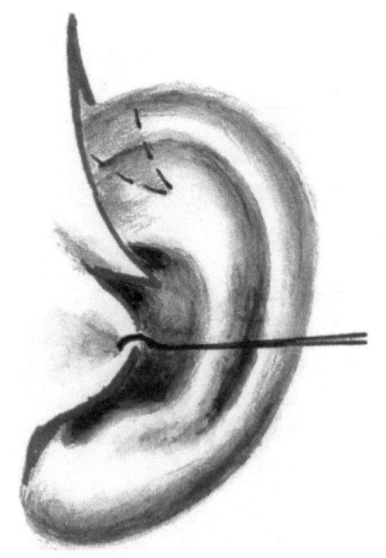
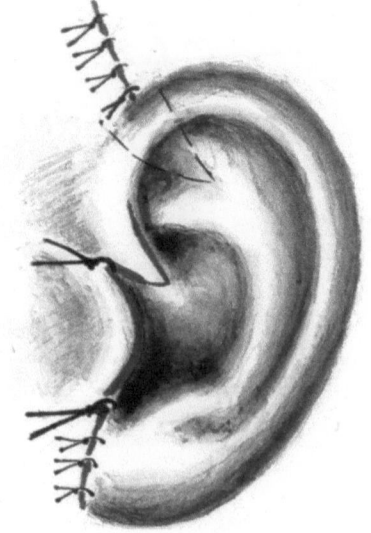

Figure 154 **Figure 155**

The details depend on the surgeon's ability not only to reproduce them but also to avoid the deep sculpting that has uncertain long-term results. The ability to insinuate the shape that produces the necessary shadows that blend to join details depends on the surgeon's experience in reconstruction and in postoperative care, until final and late results can be evaluated.

Absent Tragus

The absent tragus has been referred to previously by this author,* with various lifting flaps to obtain finer tragus results. It is advisable to avoid the Kirkham[2] method, so that the conchal floor can be preserved for canal extension.

My previous methods have been combined and modified, with tissue brought in from adjacent areas by using a large lobule as a free composite graft or swung up as an island flap pedicled on the anterior ramus of the anterior auricular vessels. A large contralateral lobule has been used as a composite graft (Fig. 156). Skin and subcutaneous tissue have also been used as an island pedicled on the anterior superficial temporal artery and veins, to transfer forehead skin and subcutaneous tissue for tragus formation. Figure 157 demonstrates a case of composite lobule to tragus graft.

Late Deepening of the Helical Sulcus

Very rarely the helical sulcus still remains too shallow. The following method has proven satisfactory to deepen it.

---

*Davis, JE. *Aesthetic and Reconstructive Otoplasty.* Springer-Verlag; 1987.

Figure 156

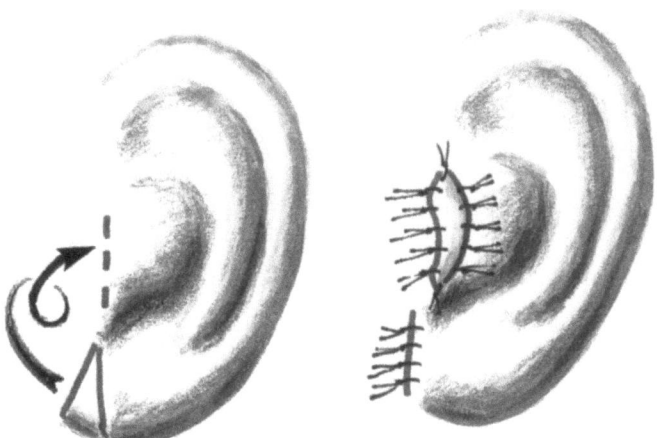

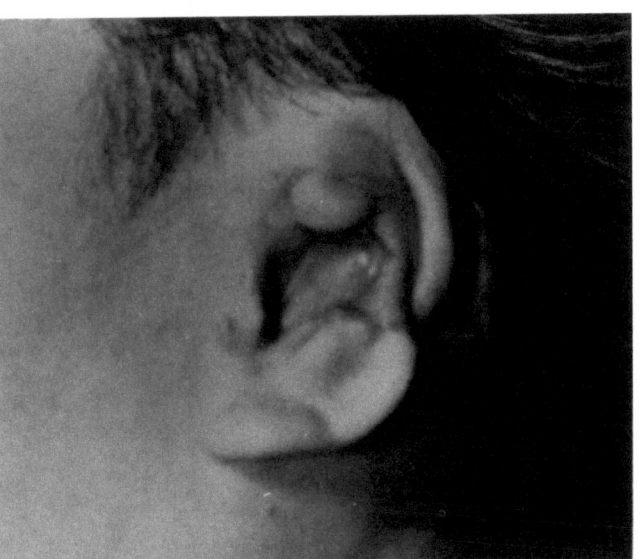

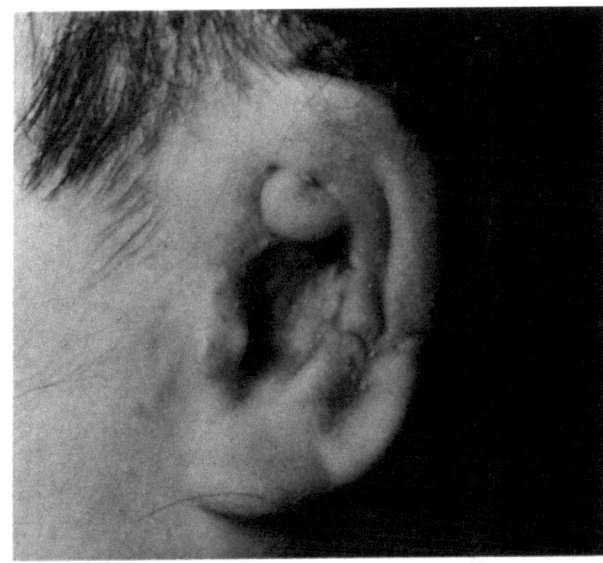

Figure 157

Figure 158 denotes the area with the collection of subcutaneous tissue, shown by shading slightly behind and above the shallow helical sulcus. The incision is skin deep, and the borders are dissected as skin thickness flaps on either side, to the limit of the lined area, up to the border of the anthelical projection, and thus also to accentuate the anthelix. Then the area is radically defatted until the grafted cartilage remains bare, as shown in Figure 158.

The anthelical cauda occasionally needs some cartilage shaving to get appropriate definition in the lower helical sulcus.

Figure 158 illustrates the manner of suturing. Inversion sutures hold the skin borders inward, and are tied over a sponge bolus. The sutures are removed in 1 month, when the helical and scaphal scar is firm.

Figure 158

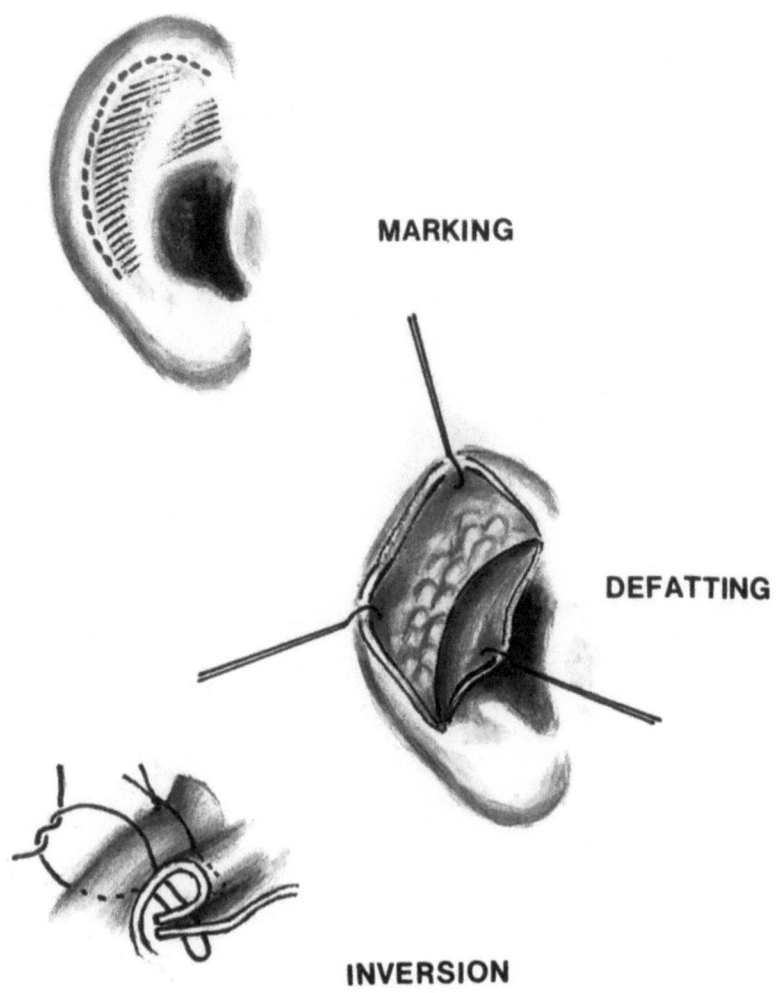

SMAS

After carefully removing the cartilaginous mass, a layer of muscle-fat remains covering the mastoid. This layer is the auricular SMAS. Occasionally, it has been used to pronounce the anthelix, by dissecting a full-thickness flap of it (Fig. 159) pedicled above and behind. The mastoid surface is bared under the mastoid fascia, thus raising the flap. The anterior flap border is then tailored and inrolled over the mastoid surface. The position is held with transfixion sutures surfaced within the hairline and tied over a bolus.

The sculpted cartilaginous frame is then placed, as usual, under the skin flap, and finally the defect is covered with a thick split-thickness skin graft, accentuating the conchal depth.

Total Auricular Atresia

In total auricular atresia the juxtatympanic pouch does not form, and the area is invaded with cancellous bone. Sometimes there is a superficial skin pit or dimple of a few millimeters' depth, but it has no connection with the deeper structures. Along the theoretical canal area cartilaginous and bony vestiges have been observed, and the bony fragments are seen in the computed tomography scans.

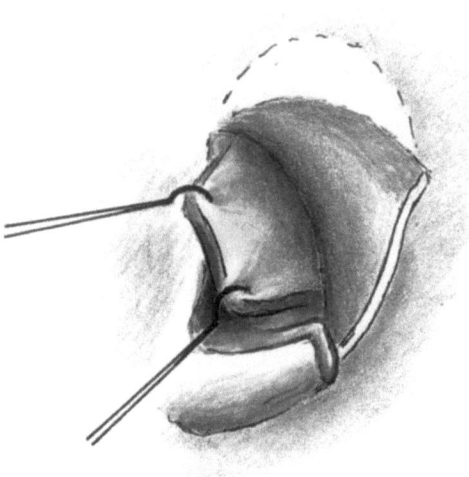
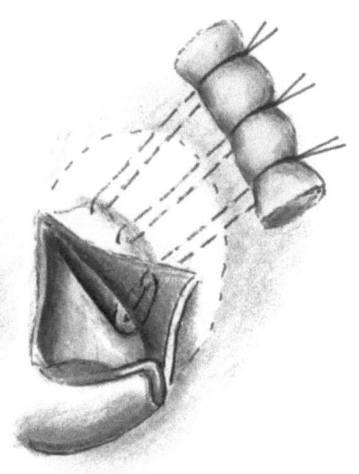

Figure 159

A careful physical examination is indicated. The type and size of the microtia is an important reference point. The symmetry and size of each mastoid is established. In general, a small mastoid is a sign of poor pneumatization, but a well-developed mastoid implies satisfactory pneumatization.

The tympanic bone and the tympanic ring are peculiar formations. The bone has no muscle or ligament insertion, and therefore is not influenced by the strain or stress of traction or pressure. It has no important organ pressing on it to give it shape. Bone condensation from stria or trabeculae is not observed. The anatomy is variable and differs from other cranial bones. The only function seems to be to sustain the tympanic membrane and keep that section of the canal open. But with no tympanic pouch formation, the tympanic bone grows without hindrance or restraint, and extends and deeply condenses to form the tympanic atresic plate.

The atresic plate has not yet been adequately defined in the literature. Exactly how it forms immediately outside the tympanic cavity has not been full explained. Understanding abnormal tympanic membrane formation is vital. The prevailing conception of "plug" resorption refers only to the canal. Considering ossification of the membrane to be secondary is incorrect. We have observed and established, to the contrary, that there is a primary insufficient mesodermic formation, with primary ossification invading the unformed area as a "waterfall." The atresic plate develops as a bony layer. This layer is later influenced superficially by resorption of the canal plug, with mass ossification from the canal cartilage, closing it as an atresia. But other tympanic bones can also form around the atresia.

Abnormal tympanic ossification is thus threefold: (1) the atresic plate, (2) the canal cartilage atresia, and (3) the supranumerary tympanic bones. The tympanic bones can be surrounded by a layer of poor condensation with cartilage remaining as a vestige along a plane of incomplete coalescence that makes it dissectable during surgery, as observed in the Davis syndrome. Later pneumatization of the middle ear presses on the atresic plate, condensing its deep surface.

Good pneumatization forms a thinner and harder plate, but poor pneumatization creates a thicker and more irregular deep plate surface.

The atresic plate's extension is variable, but it always covers the tympanic cavity. Its edges extend and feather into the surrounding bones without demarcation, from eburnated to cancellous, scaling in modality from the tympanic plate to the mastoid and zygoma below and the squama above. The deep surface of the atresic plate adheres to the tympanic cavity mucosa, which has been well observed embryologically and is important for surgery. This deep atresic plate bony surface is irregular, and varies from case to case. But the most important surgical factor is that the mucosa is always sufficiently differentiated to allow dissection from the bony plate.

Dissection is exacting, but with patience and precision a well-vascularized mucosa layer can be cleanly detached from the bone, and preserved to obtain a good surface for skin grafting.

The malleus has been observed to be adherent to the plate, but there is usually a plane of division between the two.

Precise diagnosis of the plate's characteristics is of surgical importance, and its thickness and extension should be carefully evaluated and measured with preoperative CT scanning. The plate is the axis of entry to the tympanic cavity. It is the guiding formation for meatomyringoplasty. The most direct access to the middle ear must be studied with HRCT scanning. It is along the tympanic remains and with this examination that the anterior approach has been established, immediately above and behind the temporomandibular joint.

The nerviducts are carefully noted for facial nerve aberrations, and the findings measured and recorded. Aerodynamic development of the mastoid cells and middle ear, however, is no indication for the mastoid posterior approach. It is merely a sign of middle ear development. During surgery, burring should avoid the mastoid cells, which are of different embryonic origin and pathology.

The advantages and disadvantages of the anterior approach have been compared with the classic posterior approach from mastoid to attic. Senior otologists have generally used the posterior route, and have diagnosed ossicular conditions that way. The anterior approach has been criticized in that it will lead to dysfunction of the temporomandibular (TM) joint by thinning the posterior articular wall. If surgery is performed as described below, this wall remains unaffected. A further objection has been the limited space of the osseous pyramid for ample canal construction. The pyramid is shaped by the TM joint, dura mater, and sinus lateralis. Vicente Diamante has contributed a radical step forward, expanding the pyramid with a bone graft, as will be discussed below.

Surgery

Meatomyringoplasty

After the conchal scoop-out at the first operation, the mastoid periosteum remains visible behind and above the TM joint. The area of osteotomy is marked, and the periosteum incised, elevated, and retracted toward the TM joint, so that the bone surface remains bare. A layer of cortical bone is then removed with a gouge size chosen to fit the case. The bone is removed in one piece to be used as a graft. This bone graft is sculpted to fit on to the TM surface, which is prepared by detaching and raising the area periosteum, and sliding the bone graft into the slot, thus extending the pyramid, as designed (Fig. 129).

This bone graft is insufficient when the pyramid is very small, and then the method developed by Diamante is used. It consists of inserting a larger bone graft taken from the mastoid apex. Four to six months later the bone graft has become firmly consolidated, and the pyramid area has been increased enough to construct an adequately calibered, canal. In this way, the second stage is prepared at the first operation, but controlled with HRCTs before going in the second time.

Although the second operation consists essentially of raising the auricle from the head with a retroaural skin graft, my aim is to construct the canal also at the same stage. About 4 months after the first operation, the soft tissue has healed well, swelling has subsided, and the bone graft has become consolidated.

Ossification is as yet untrabeculated and easy to trephine. The periosteum has formed a cortical layer that has to be removed, but the canal area is amplified. At this second operation, after finishing the auricle, the canal is approached. The area to be drilled is prepared, and the microscope is brought in, as well as the nerve stimulator.

Stereotactic Surgery

Oscar Candás (otosurgeon), José Rosler (neurosurgeon), and I have developed a new and very useful surgical maneuver for construction of the external aural canal in congenital ear atresia, diminishing both operation time and the number of operations for the reconstruction. The plastic surgeon marks the exact position of the surface mastoid approach for the canal to coincide with auricular repair. The canal can then be made with the following conditions:

1. Precision point of entry to the mastoid cortex is marked with an indentation.
2. It allows exact calculation of the target point over the middle ear, without unnecessary vibration and preserving the tympanic mucosa.
3. Thus, the least possible mastoid cells are opened.
4. The temporomandibular joint is not exposed.
5. The dura is not reached.
6. The facial nerve or its rami are avoided.
7. The canal should be large enough to obtain good function, with adequate ossicular observation.
8. But be narrow enough to avoid creating a mastoid cavity that can become diseased in originally healthy tissue.

The obvious advantage of the anterior approach is that it is the most direct, shortest, and most perpendicular route to the middle ear. It allows

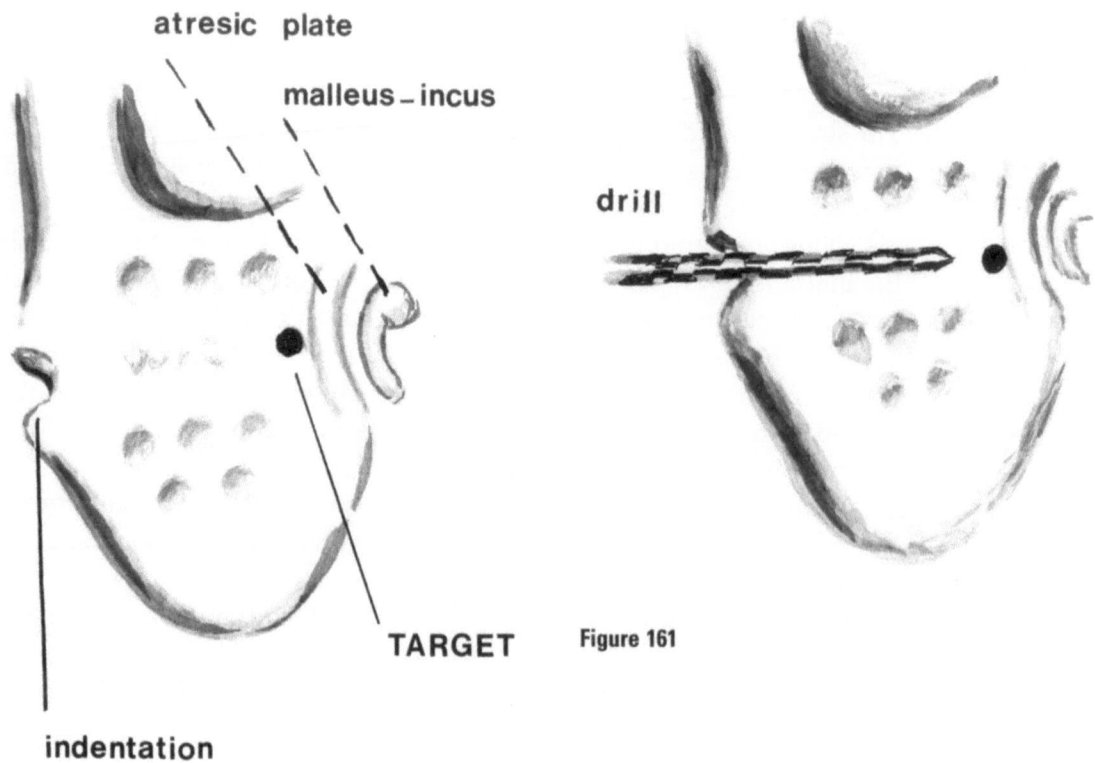

Figure 160

Figure 161

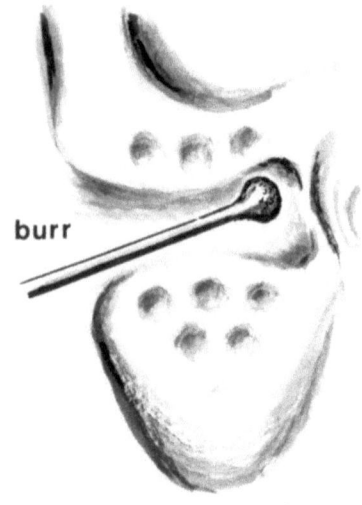

Figure 162

observation of the malleus, stapes, fenestra, and the relationship between the atresic plate and the malleus. It has had the best results in our experience.

The plastic surgeon raises a conchal skin flap and bares the mastoid. He then indents the bone exactly where the canal should be with relation to the auricle he has reconstructed (Fig. 160). Precise positioning of auricle and canal is the key to the combined approach. The proper direction of entry after the surface indentation has not always been adequate. With stereotactic computation and facial nerve monitoring it becomes exactly precise with a 3-mm drill and slow motor (Fig. 161). Drilling is deepened to 2 mm from the middle ear mucosa, reaching the atresic plate surface, to reach the target point.

The 3-mm perforation guide is then expanded with otologic burs (Fig. 162). The canal shape is normally not cylindrical, but mildly hourglass. The external auditory canal is wider at the surface than in the depth. The narrower central part is called the isthmus and is located about 19 mm from the conchal floor surface in the adult. We have carefully shaped the meatus with a gently curved surface from conchal floor to canal, and avoided a sharp, square, step deformity between the two, tapering smoothly for the best aesthetics and function, and to achieve easy cleaning.

Magnetic resonance imaging with a superficial coil, computed tomography, and audiometric tests are used to determine facial nerve aberrations, which are common in this deformity, and to position the middle ear.

We have used a stereotactic guide to reach the 3D target point at the mid-atresic plate, approaching the tympanic mucosa and close to the lateral ossicle. The procedure commences with skull fixation (Fig. 164) of the

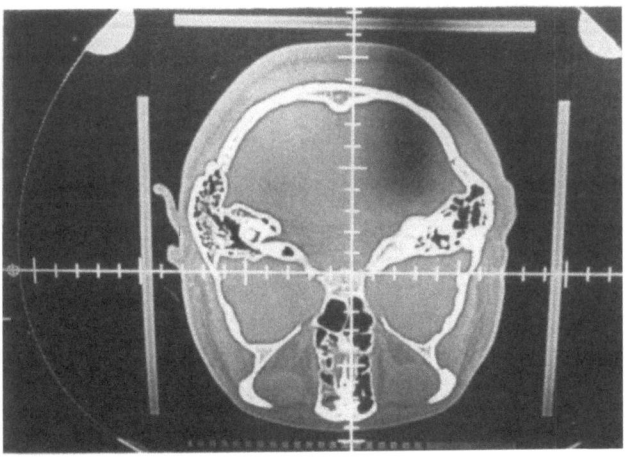
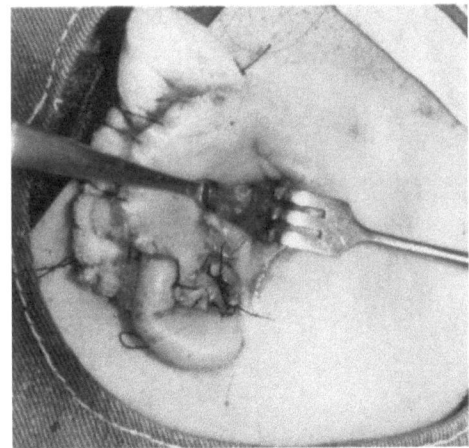

Figure 163

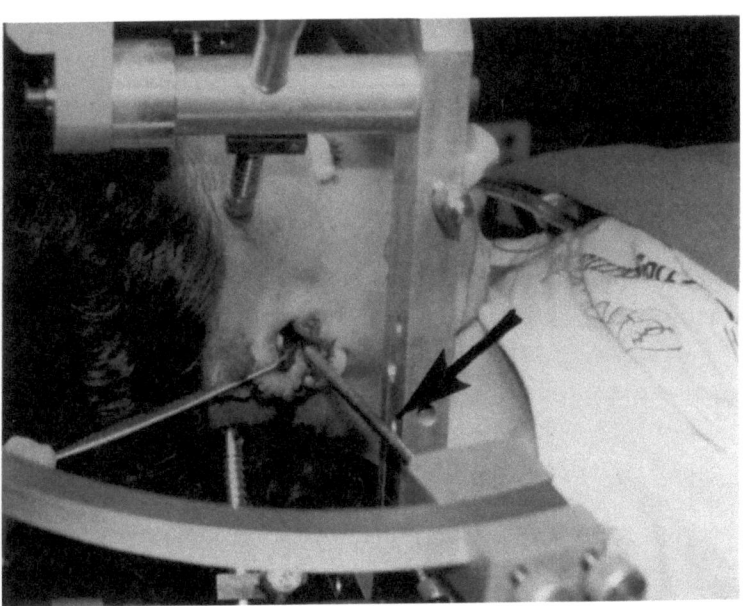
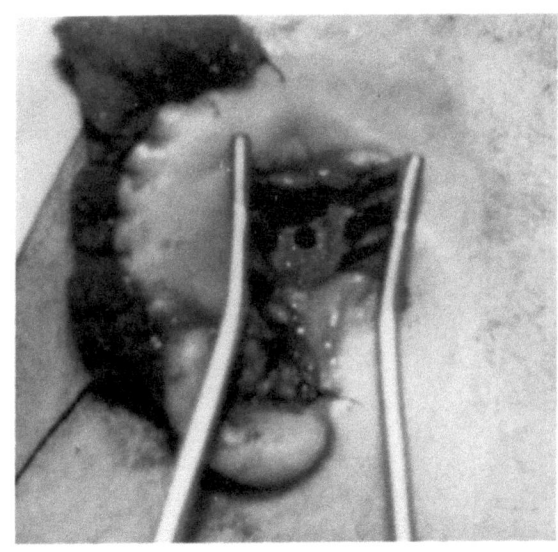

Figure 164

stereotactic frame, under neuroleptoanalgesia. An HRCT scan is taken under stereotactic conditions (Fig. 163), which allow precise targeting. This maneuver provides the shortest and most direct approach to the atresic plate without unnecessary exploration. It directs the otosurgeon's burs for amplification.

The mastoid surface is bared during the second stage, after the postauricular sulcus had been deepened and skin-grafted. The stereotactic frame is firmly attached to the cranium (Fig. 164). The arrow indicates the drill shaft. The resulting 3 mm diameter perforation guides the otosurgeon's approach.

The tympanic atresic bone may be cancellous, cortical, or fragmented, but it has to be removed to uncover the atresic plate lateral surface, led by the pathway previously mapped out, avoiding the facial nerve or nerves positioned by HRCT and controlled with neurostimulation, and keeping close to the TM joint. The deeper canal is expanded to shape the juxtatympanic pouch on reaching the atresic plate.

Surgery

A normal external auditory canal caliber is between 9.8 and 8.3 mm maximum and 6.45 and 4.60 minimum. Average canal length is 24 mm, of which 8 mm is fibrocartilaginous and 16 mm osseous. The canal space can be judged to be the size of the distal little finger.

The whole lateral surface of the atresic plate is entirely uncovered, which is usually a circle of about 10 mm diameter. Only a diamond bur is used, and it is kept cool. Heat will destroy both the graft and the recipient surface, and must be absolutely avoided. Once the plate is bare, drilling is performed with great care (Fig. 165). The diamond bur will eat the bone away but not the soft tissue. The atresic plate is gradually reduced in thickness until becoming transparent. A violet hue appears in places reaching the mucosa, and with tiny perforations the bone edges are rasied with the hooks and curette technique to fracture them toward the surface, as performed in the fenestration technique (Fig. 166).

When this has been done with maximum care, it is possible to keep the underlying tissue intact (Fig. 167). It has been found that the underlying mucosa is not even, due to irregularities of the bone surface that had to be followed. If the malleus manubrium forms part of the atresic plate, it is removed. But if it is included in the mucosa and is independent of the plate, which is usually the case, it is dissected attached to the mucosa. When there is a good-functioning eustachian tube, the mucosa balloons out with expiration and is sucked in with inspiration. When the mucosa surface has been cleared and all adhesions removed, the condition of the malleus is carefully observed transparently through the lining of the middle ear, and the malleus-incus synostosis and stapes are examined for chain continuity and their movement is explored by manipulating them. We think that the skin graft laid on an intact mucosa with mobile ossicles is the secret of success at this stage.

Figure 165

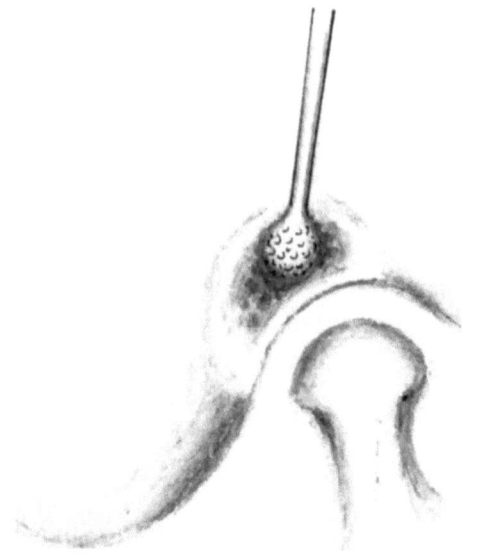

Figure 166

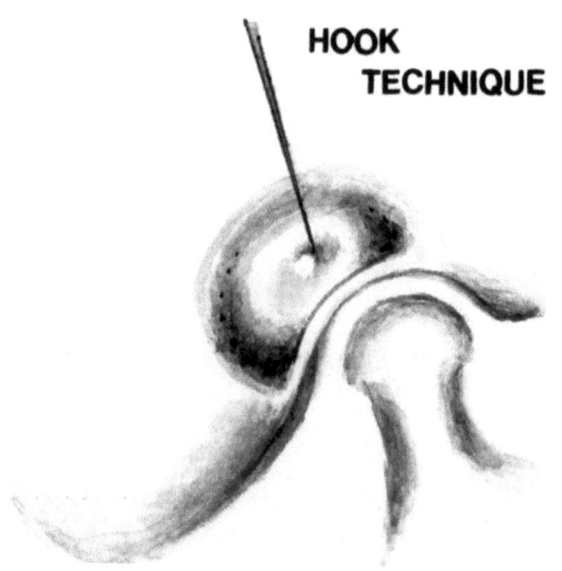

Figure 167

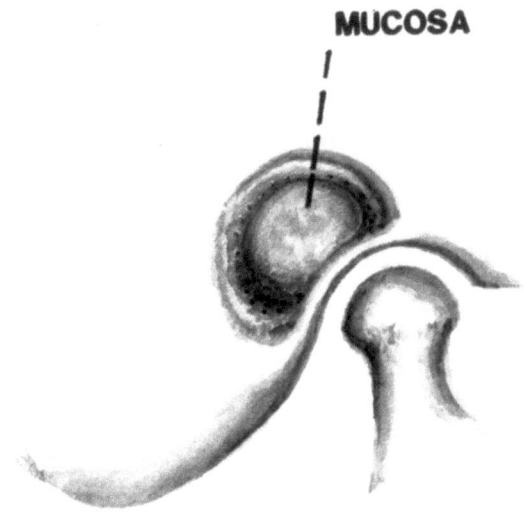

Figure 168

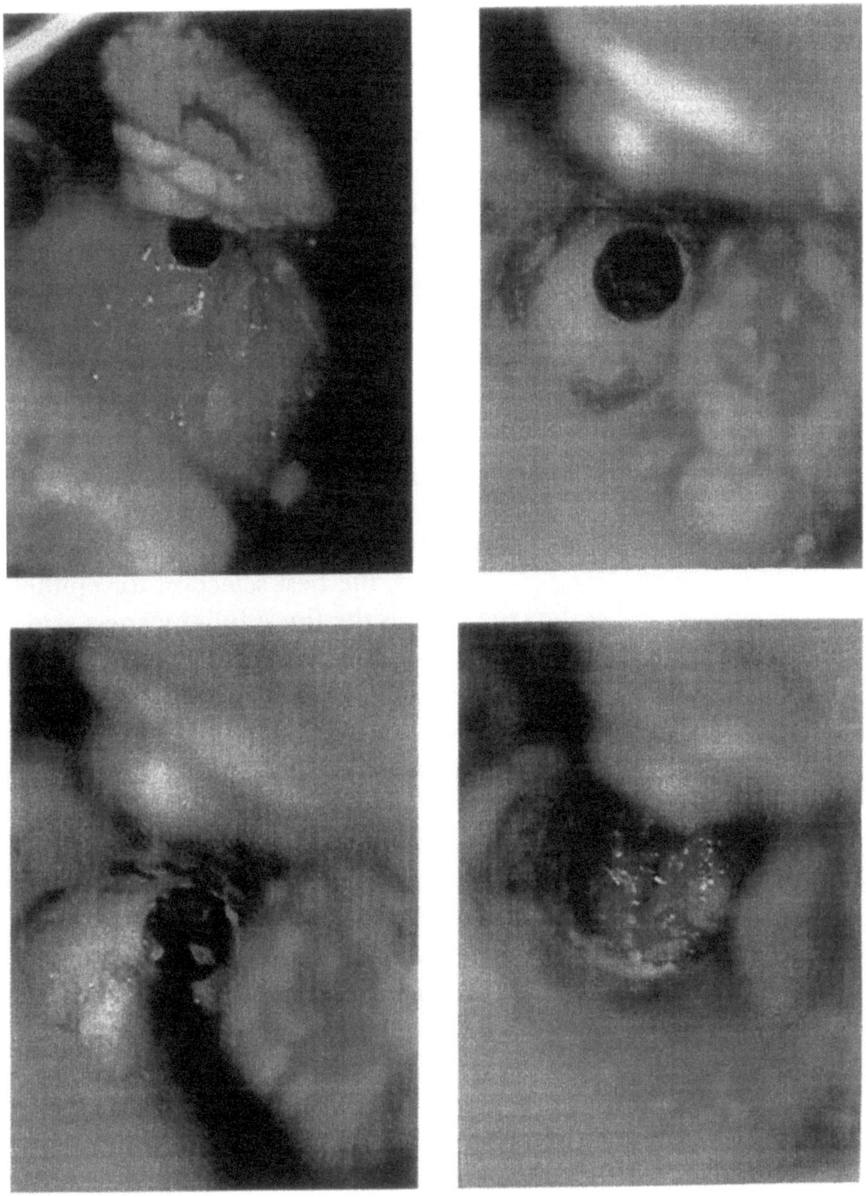

Surgery

The microphotographs show (Fig. 168): stereotactic perforation and amplification of the canal and the result of the curette and hook technique of the atresic plate. Ossicles are observed through the intact mucosa. The mucosa is ready to receive the skin graft. All adhesions and bony connection with the ossicles are removed.

Covering the Neotympanic Membrane

Due to the importance of this covering, insistence on some details can be of value. The skin graft has to be ample enough to receive sound waves, elastic enough to allow adequate transmission of sound, and easy enough for the patient to clean. The patient should not be reduced to being a permanent invalid, dependent permanently on the surgeon who did the job. Who else will continue cleaning the intricate and multidetailed canals? Also, the next surgeon cannot possibly know all the details. Therefore, the reconstructed canals must be ample enough, as short as possible, beveled toward the surface with a mild cone shape, with even, smooth walls, without hair or excess desquamation. The patient must be able to easily clean the canal by syringing with soap and water.

Thick skin grafts, which are taken from the thigh or buttock, simply fill the canal lumen. "Thick" applies not only to the graft per se but also to the added desquamation. "Thin" grafts usually refer to partial-thickness grafts taken from the medial arm respect. The obvious inconvenience is the retraction, both from the graft border and the bed fibrosis. When the graft retracts, it becomes tense and stiff. Retraction in a circular tube is far greater than on a flat surface. Even very fine split-thickness grafts will grow hair from the intradermal follicules. The scars will retract. The thinner the graft, the greater the retraction.

Flaps have been considered and tried, but they are simply too bulky for deep canal work. Local flaps can be well used, however, for superficial reconstruction of the canal.

Thus, the best selection for epithelial lining of the deeper section of the canal is the finest full-thickness skin grafts possible. The finest are from the upper eyelid, but the available surface is insufficient in relatively young patients. The answer is skin of transition with mucosa of sufficient surface. It does not grow hair, it is ideally soft, flexible, and elastic, and is to be found in the prepuce penis foreskin in the male; equally useful has been the skin of transition of the labia majoris in the female. There is enough skin to cover the neotympanic area to excess, and curl up over the wall without plications of irregularities until the deeper canal has been covered.

The wider superficial meatus of the canal, however, needs a different texture of epithelium. Thicker skin grafts, preferably from the mastoid area combined with local fine flaps brought in from the concha, have worked best. It is important to stagger the suture lines to avoid circular scar retraction.

These principles have proven true in practice, and good results have been obtained. The necessary difference of lining of the two canal sections has been well reproduced (Fig. 169). The deep is covered with fine, flexi-

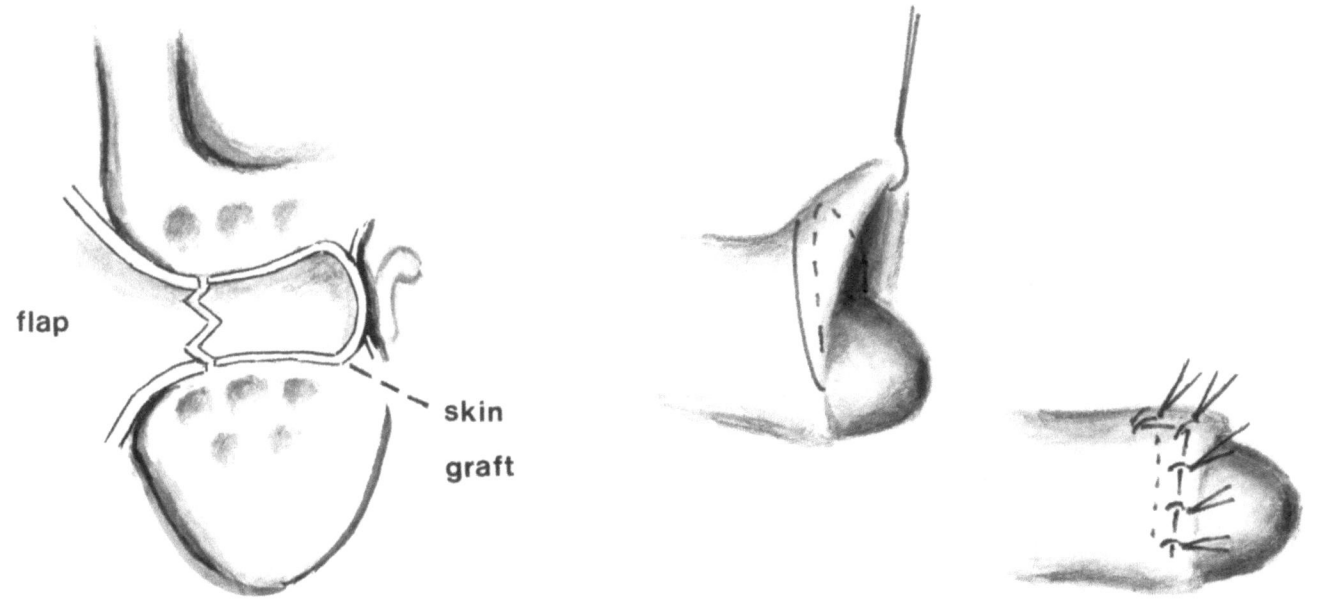

Figure 169   Figure 170

ble, elastic, hairless, and glandless skin over the neotympanic and juxtatympanic area, while the canal meatus is covered with fine flaps that bear downy hairs and ceruminous glands, and that recover with nervous reflex defense ability.

Obtaining the necessary caliber, with a smooth, even canal surface and staggered scars, is the surgeon's challenge and goal.

There are some details about the manner of prepuce skin graft removal that are worth mentioning (Fig. 170). This is delicate epithelium that is best removed as illustrated. Closure of the donor wound is staggered with a dorsal Z-plasty to relax the finally incomplete circular scar, and preserve enough loose skin for normal erection.

The quantity of skin removed must be sufficient to cover the neotympanic and adjacent surfaces. The skin graft is meticulously prepared as a full-thickness graft, and carefully cleaned of all fat and fascia until the basal membrane is bare.

By suturing the prepuce graft to the conchal flap over a fingertip, with the skin raw surface inward and keeping the strands long, a "bag" is shaped (Figs. 171 and 172). Then the bag is turned inside-out, so that the raw surfaces of both flap and graft remain outward. The bag is placed in the canal lodge, carefully adapting the graft over the mucosa under the microscope. The sutures remain within the bag. The skin is covered with Vaseline gauze and the cavity is lightly packed with sponge pellets. The pellets are removed in 12 days.

It is routine for otosurgeons to use temporalis fascia as a free graft spread over the exposed middle ear elements, and to cover it with a skin graft. Success depends on a secondary mucose border closure that will advance over a small area. But a larger area will remain with incomplete revascularization of the two grafts, fascia and skin, and a central ulceration and

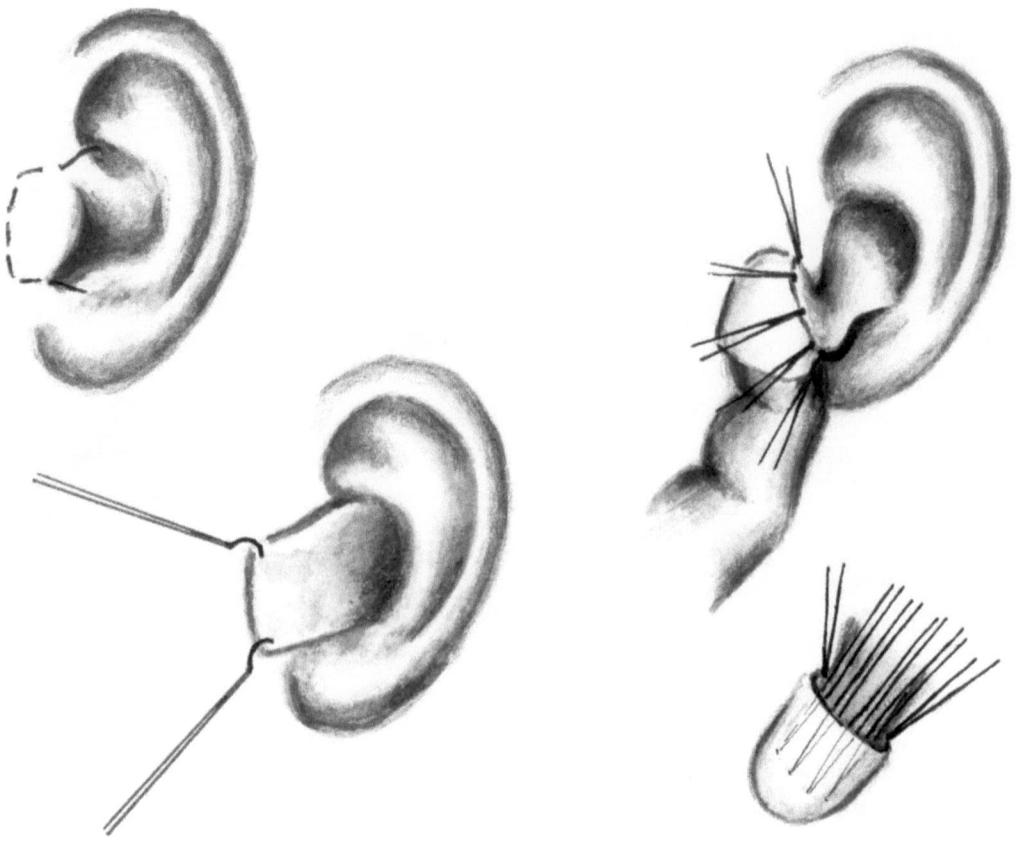

Figure 171

Figure 172

fistulae will ensue. The fistulae remain as a red spot growing and everted tympanic cavity mucosa. Overlaid grafts go against plastic surgery principles and should be avoided. Although full-thickness skin has given ideal results, with adequate precision fine medial arm split-thickness skin (not withstanding previously mentioned limitations) can give excellent results if carefully used.

It is important that the graft be one undivided sheet, considerably larger than the area to be covered, as designed (Fig. 173). The canal is drilled larger than is finally needed, allowing for retraction. The graft is deepened into a clean canal lodge, devoid of bleeding by prolonged compression. Fairly large plastic sponge cubes hold the depth so that the graft is in close contact with the mucosa. More sponge cubes fill the cavity. To avoid the sponges becoming adhered to the skin grafts, antiseptic Vaseline gauze strips are placed immediately over the skin, allowing easy removal of the sponges in 6 to 7 postoperative days.

The graft borders must overlap the meatus border flaps, held by a few anchoring sutures. Further transfixion sutures are tied over a larger superficial sponge to hold the rest in place, as a tie-on dressing.

Surgery is easier when done on patients older than 6 years of age. The demand for adequate function of the auricle and canal are the present measure. Both aspects, aesthetic and functional, are considered. Auricular cartilage framework solves most drawbacks. Why did the healing potential im-

Figure 173

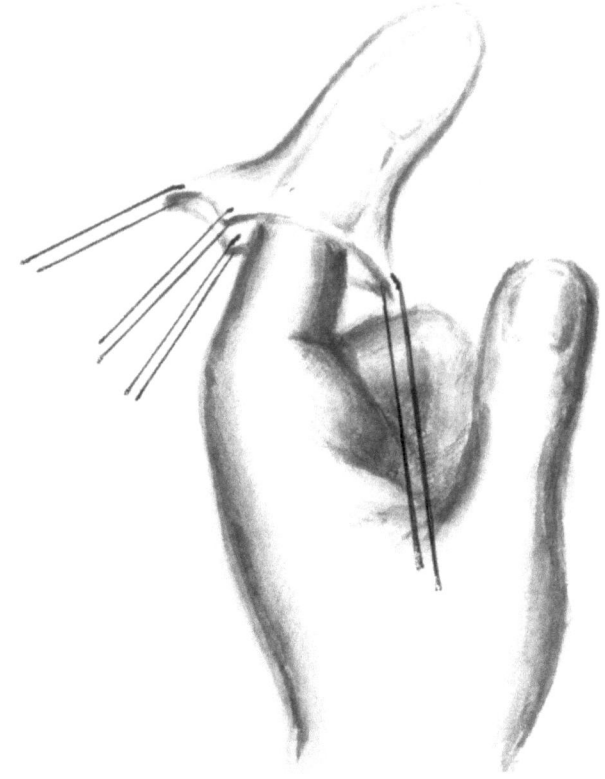

prove so radically? Second-intention healing has been spontaneous. Granulation tissue formation and epithelialization without cartilage loss has not needed plastic maneuvers to cover the frame. The probable explanation is that the auricular graft was covered with perichondrium on both surfaces, which readily attract vascularization. Blood, lymph, and nerve ingrowth occur via the perichondrium. The minimal pseudocapsular formation and the auricular muscle reinsertion undoubtedly play a part and facilitate the anterior canal approach. The hinge maneuver, raising the rigid pinna of costal cartilage frame and retracting it forward to approach the mastoid bone retroaurally, should be avoided.

No discussion has been found in the medical literature about using the stereotactic technique for congenital microtia and atresia, but although it has been most useful in our experience, no mechanical device can replace the knowledge and dexterity of a good surgeon.

Thus, the following points for meatomyringoplasty have been established:

1. The shortest, most direct approach to the middle ear in atresia, avoiding the facial nerve and mastoid cells, is the anterior approach.
2. The canal must have adequate shape, size, caliber, and positioning for the tympanic membrane.
3. The neotympanic membrane should be closely adapted to mobile connected ossicles.

4. The neotympanic membrane should be sufficiently elastic, flexible, and mobile.
5. The middle ear lining should be salvaged.
6. Open, wide exploratory middle ear surgery and tympanoplastic maneuvers should be avoided when possible.
7. Keep the air bubble, to care for normal mastoid-tube drainage.
8. Obtain a "dry" result.
9. Only estimate results after 10 months. Earlier controls are during the inflammatory period of healing and are only transitory observations.
10. Instruct the patient to clean the canal.
11. Reeducate the patient's hearing by training him or her to use the new organ.
12. The underlying concept that governs canal reconstruction in total atresia is that auriculoplasty should not be a solitary procedure. The auricle and canal are an anatomical and functional unit, but the auricle repair precedes the meatomyringoplasty.
13. The atresia is not corrected simply by making a skin-lined hole, but rather by complying with all the requirements of functional repair.

Results

Meatomyringoplasty results have varied. The best have been with the method described, but every case is different, and much depends on the capacity of the patient to use the new organ. It has been common to obtain social hearing, but with the precision of the method described, close to normal hearing has been acquired.

Early audiometric tests are not useful. They should only be considered after healing is complete (usually at 1 year). Even the reossification can appear years later. Audiometry is a relative measure of results. Audiostereognosis is an important component to be considered. Many other deeper aural functions that are still under investigation further extend the sphere of otologic evaluation and are becoming gradually better known in otology. However, we have been impressed by the overall satisfaction of our patients with otologic improvement, which has definitely made this surgery worthwhile.

The measure of results should refer only to the meatomyringoplasty as the combined work of the plastic surgeon and otosurgeon. Middle and even internal ear abnormalities have to be considered when evaluating auditory acuity. Especially chain discontinuity and stapes fixation have usually caused a more severe conduction hearing loss that can be estimated with preoperative audiograms and HRCTs, and during surgery with chain movement examination. But tympanotomy and tympanoplasty are best postponed, to be considered when meatomyringoplasty healing has been completed after 1 year. If late otologic controls indicate further surgery, I believe that tympanotomy and tympanoplasty should remain entirely within the domain of the otosurgeon who has specialized in this field.

Sometimes I have been surprised with results of total canal repair. One patient even surpassed the normal audiometric range. Her parents were embarrassed when she could hear what they were whispering at the other side of the room. She herself found that mass sound perception was uncomfortable. With time, she gradually discriminated and balanced sound perception, and after 1 year she was no longer uncomfortable.

Another patient obtained exceptionally good hearing, but she did not respond when she was not looking straight at me. I only then realized the importance of audiometry, because she was secretly an expert lip reader.

Secondary Strictures

Little has been published about late strictures of the reconstructed canal, but they seem to have been experienced by every surgeon devoted to this work. In reviewing our cases and others, it was possible to divide these strictures into two types: superficial and deep. The superficial strictures were due to soft tissue defects from scars or grafts that were related to the surgery, and usually occurred during the first postoperative year.

But when the defect was deep, it was due to bone reforming, appeared later (frequently 3 years or more), and was more difficult to repair. Reossification had occurred from three sources:

1. Normal mastoid growth in children, toward the area of least resistance.
2. Subperiosteum osteogenesis of the deep canal, especially around the neotympanic membrane. Therefore, the periosteum must be carefully removed for the tympanum, but the mucosa preserved for reconstruction.
3. Porous endosteum reossification of the midcanal, as in any mastoid fracture.

These three mechanisms can combine, or one can be dominant. Both careful otologic examination and detailed HRCTs are necessary. Late strictures have to be considered individually, calculating the healing potential of the patient. The best time to reoperate is when area growth has finished and results are stable, usually at 18 years of age. The repaired canal should be slightly larger than virgin cases, to calculate for a certain degree of contracture. The shape needs to be deeply cylindrical but tapering as a cone wider toward the surface, so it should eventually be easy to clean.

The following case describes late findings in a patient originally operated on for ear repair and meatomyringoplasty at 6 years of age. The canal gradually closed throughout the years and is shown at 19 years of age. The patient was found to have a mixed-type reossification. The following microphotographs, taken during surgery (Fig. 174) show a horizontal hemicircumferential approach, with a horizontal L meatal extension, removal of many curious little bony balls, the size of gunshot pellets, surrounded by dense fibrous tissue, amplification of the canal with the bur, and the preserved vascularized skin flaps, which were enough to cover the new surface without the need of adding further skin grafts.

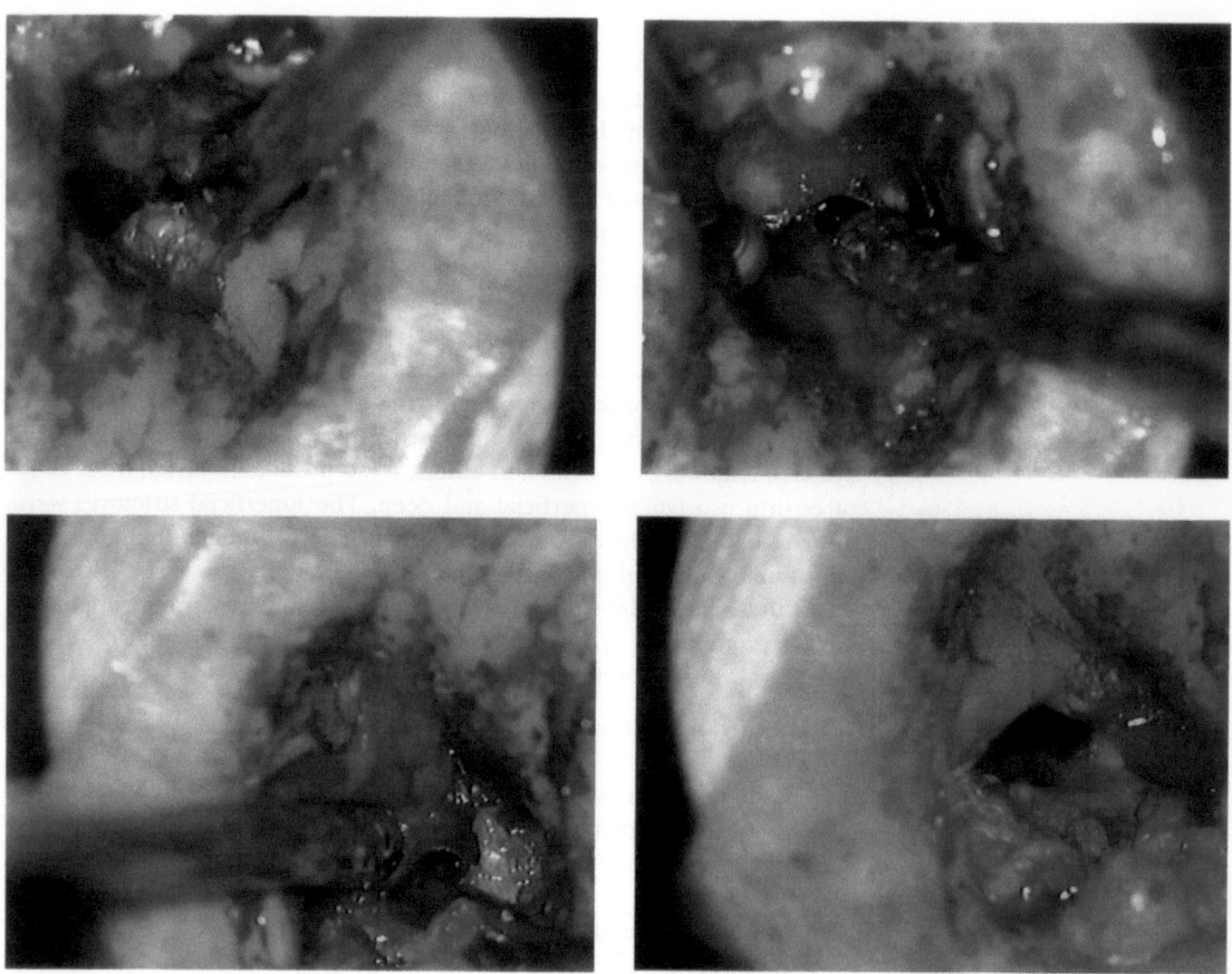

Figure 174

Result

The retroaural sulcus has been deepened and skin grafted during the same operation.

6
Bilateral Microtia and Atresia

Unilateral microtia and atresia have been statistically demonstrated to have been satisfactorily repaired using autogenous auricular cartilage. The key question is: How about bilateral cases? This is quite a different sphere, but the basic principles remain:

1. Auricular cartilage is not duplicated elsewhere in the body.
2. The ideal material for microtia repair is autogenous ear material, which paves the way for myringoplasty.
3. Microtia and atresia are one entity, to be reconstructed together.

Attempted auricular repair with homo- and necro-grafts and allogen material (silicone, etc.), have failed in the long term, which precludes them from consideration. As the current choice for framework material is sculpted costal cartilage, rib cartilage must now be evaluated, establishing advantages and drawbacks. The advantage is that the final shape has improved in the hands of a few sculptor surgeons, who have beautifully photographed their work with excellent shape and color.

Other factors, apart from shape and color, should be considered in classifying a human organ and in aiming for ideal results.

The drawbacks of costal cartilage are the following:

1. Donor site thoracotomy, with occasional danger of pleural complications. Perforation and rupture from anomalous or pathologic pleural adhesions, pneumothorax, and pleuricy have been reported.
2. Chest wall deformities after chondrectomy. I have managed to mitigate the chest wall depression by returning all sculpted cartilage flakes back into the original lodge that filled the void with a chondrofibrous mass. However, this method has not met with general acclaim, and repeated final surgical chest deformities have been reported.
3. The chest deformity, leaves an unnecessary and unsightly scar, and frequently is evident because it does not fall exactly into the area's skin tension lines.
4. Prolonged hospitalization and its cost, as well as the cost of the major surgery (thoracotomy).
5. Costal cartilage is hyaline tissue that normally becomes rigid, calcified, and even osseous. It never loses the tendency to progressive

rigidity, and it becomes hard and even brittle with time. This has been demonstrated embryologically, histopathologically, and clinically. When costal cartilage is grafted, this process is faster. As a graft, it is not invaded by blood or lymph vessels or ingrowing nerve supply. Area neurologic reestablishment is late and limited. The graft becomes surrounded by a pseudocapsule as a manner of biologic integration. This pseudocapsule is nature's way of tolerating and yet partially isolating the graft. Thus, surrounding tissues are easily peeled away from the costal graft. Trauma produces hematoma, when a rupture of the pseudocapsule takes place, and blood collects between it and the graft. As the postaural sulcus is rigid and does not give way elastically to accommodate eyeglass earpieces, the skin becomes ulcerated and requires many months of careful treatment to heal. Infection spreads easily, and then total chondritis of the frame occurs.

6. Patients become conscious of these limitations and become defensive about the reconstructed organ. One outspoken youngster asked me, "Doc, what am I going to do with this horn sticking out of my head?"

7. The lack of elasticity and flexibility, and other functions affecting the trophic healing potential, reduce the freedom of the otologic approach in space and quality. Any interference or adverse factor affecting the best conditions for simultaneous canal and auricle reconstruction must be avoided.

Auricular cartilage is quite special, and it is irreplaceable in a patient's lifetime. As I have come to learn its value, it saddens me to recall the times this wonderful tissue has been thrown away in the surgical dustbin.

Microtial cartilage is like an iceberg: most of it lies below the surface. I feel that this reconstruction should be guided by the principle that maximum use be made of available native cartilage. My idea that microtia is like a bud that needs to bloom is applied in practice. When the microtial cartilage is brought up and the petals laid out, much is obtained. I have termed this *expansion chondroplasty*, and I believe it will open a new field in radical otoplasty.

Auriculoplasty must pave the way for improving auditory acuity. Hearing loss in bilateral cases is much more important than in unilateral cases. Canal construction has been performed after auriculoplasty, as in unilateral microtia. Timing the sequence is as follows:

First operation: first-stage auriculoplasty on one side.

Second operation: second-stage auriculoplasty and canal on the same side, and first-stage auriculoplasty on the other.

Third operation: third-stage auriculoplasty and canal on the other side. The sequence commences when the patient is 6 years of age, with surgery repeated at intervals of 4 months. Detailed otologic examinations for precise diagnosis is done prior to canal and middle ear surgery. The best results are with bilateral myringoplasty and canal construction. This is the reason to postpone surgery on bilateral microtia and atresia to the age at which unilateral cases have been done, so that the child is taught the early use of hearing aids and thus avoids any learning retardment. At 6 years of age CT can be performed with less fear of x-ray damage, and the child is old enough to appropriately participate in audiometric examination.

Bilateral Atresia

Otologic Considerations

The study should commence soon after birth, to determine the degree of auditory loss and to treat the child early to avoid language impairment. From 0 to 6 months the following methods are indicated:

Observation audiometry.

Audiometric brainstem response (ABR).

Middle latency potentials (MLP).

Acoustic otoemissions.

From 6 to 12 months:

Sound localization.

Response to speech in a natural atmosphere.

ABR.

MLP.

Acoustic otoemissions.

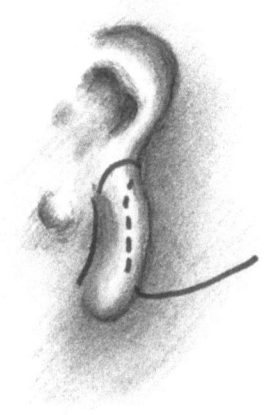

Figure 175

The child is expected to have a 60-dB bilateral deafness from conductive hearing loss. An immediate hearing aid is indicated, as a headband vibrator. The child should use this aid until surgery, which is best done when he or she is 6 years of age. As the aid is worn only on one ear, change of ear is indicated to stimulate and evaluate each one. Surgery commences with auriculoplasty, and the atresias are operated on one at a time. Preoperative HRCT is essential. No two atresias are the same.

The surgery designs show the skin incisions and the lobule setback (Fig. 175). On dissecting the lobule for the setback, all fatty trabecular tissue is kept on the flap for antitragus bulk. When positioning the flap, this excess fatty tissue is finally covered with an extension of the conchal skin graft at the first stage. The skin should be excessive to allow the extra fat to be incorporated and to increase the lobular height, and it should be made slightly more bulky to allow for retraction, but still mark the antitragus.

The microtial cartilage is removed by very careful dissection with fine scissors, and only a cartilage flake is kept in place to shape the tragus, in position and of adequate size (Fig. 176).

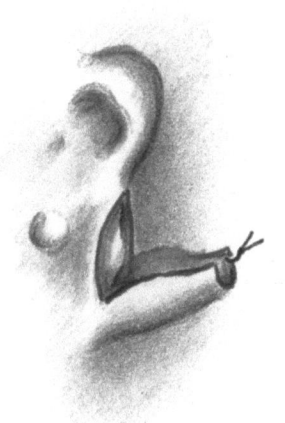

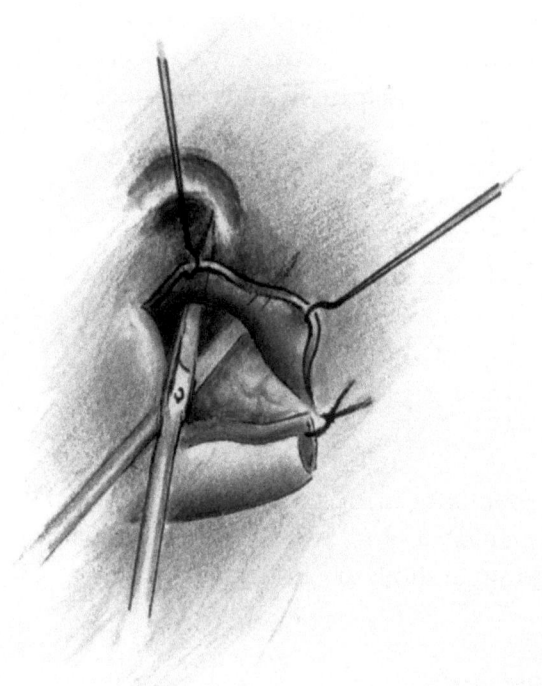

Figure 176

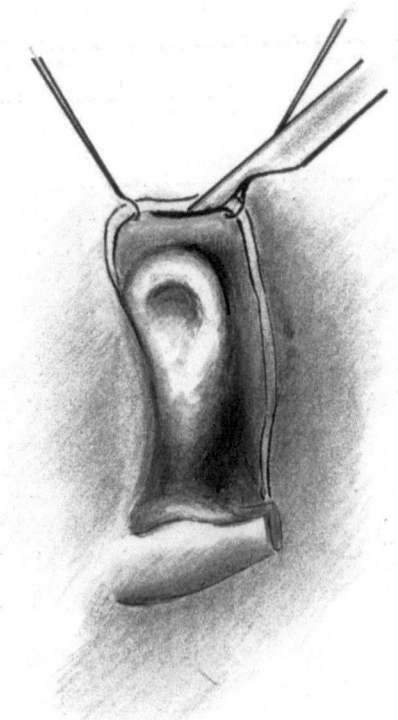

Figure 177

Upper Nubbin

The upper nubbin is special. The integument over it is unique. It would seem that the auricular dorsal skin and subcutaneous layer have extended up and over the upper microtic pole. The skin is of excellent quality for reconstruction—uniform and well vascularized. Below the skin, the fat is different from other microtial fat, and is composed of two layers divided by a fascia. The superficial fat layer is trabecular, limited, and firm, forming a pad. But the deeper layer is looser and thin, with a good plane of cleavage dissectable from the cartilage mass.

It is necessary to reach the trabecular layer by incising the fascia (Fig. 177) and then progressing immediately below the skin. Only when the skin is free can it be spread out to be plastically usable. This skin is especially useful for shaping the anterior helix, lower crus, and adjacent depressions. The fascia is usually discarded, but occasionally it is rolled and contributes to shape the anterior helix.

The anterior microtial skin, however, is pitted and closely adheres to the underlying cartilage, with scarce subcutaneous tissue, and it would seem to be malformed scaphal skin. It is of less value, and should be used with reserve in the reconstruction.

Framework

When the cartilage mass is removed, it is carefully examined. By opening and gently expanding the crumpled auricular petals, it is useful to start with a marked helical sulcus. The best instruments in my experience for this dissection are eyelid scissors and a very fine Freer elevator. Once the helical

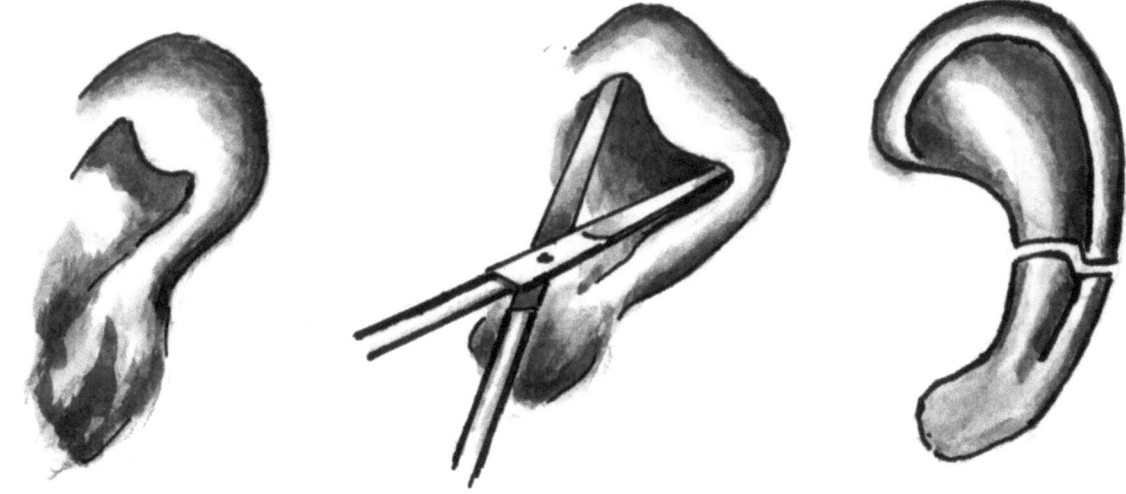

Figure 178

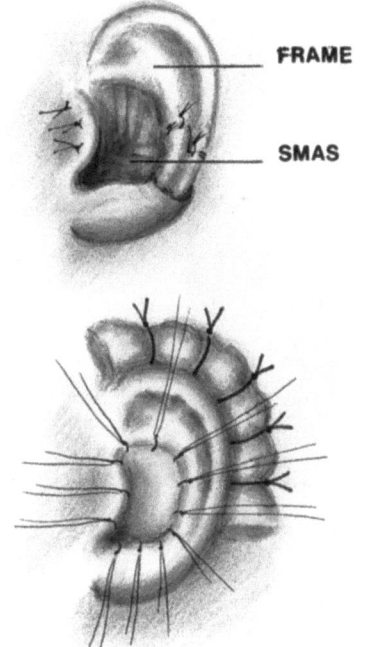

Figure 179

sulcus is shaped, the helical borders are trimmed. Then the upper scapha and superior auricular framework are formed from the remaining mass (Fig. 178).

The lower crumpled part of microtial cartilage is used to model the lower framework, which is much easier. It is remarkable how much useful microtial cartilage has been found.

Each fragment is sculpted, tailored to fit together precisely, and sutured into place with 6-0 braided silk (Fig. 179). The frame is shaped as shown and placed over the skin to gauge the ear size and shape. The SMAS layer is below. The central circle of this SMAS layer is removed to scoop out and deepen the concha, and thus provide the relief.

The SMAS contracture test (Davis method) is useful in measuring the site and quantity of muscle to be removed, and this has also been studied previously by the otosurgeon and CT radiologist, to mark the exact approach and position of the future canal toward the atresic plate. Outside the excised circle enough muscle is kept to be firmly sutured to the framework to function as normal SMAS (Fig. 179).

This expansion chondrotomy must not be confused with expansile framework as practiced by Burton Brent. The principle, mechanics, and surgery are quite different.

The frame is then inserted under the skin flap, and the cauda sutured to the lobular cartilage. The helical sulcus is pronounced by indenting it with transfixion sutures held with a bolus surfaced within the hairline. These sutures also anchor the cartilage into place.

A thick, hairless partial-thickness inguinal skin graft is set over the conchal floor and held with tie-on sutures carefully placed, piercing the four border elements (skin flap, cartilage border, SMAS, and skin graft), and knotted to hold them firmly together. The strands are kept long enough to be used later for the tie-on dressing.

The SMAS muscles attached to the frame contribute to reinnervation, trophism, later ear movement, and to anchoring the framework into place.

Framework

Bilateral microtia corrected with auricular cartilage commenced with the use of microtial cartilage from both ears to reconstruct one of them, in 1987. A patient is shown with the right side repaired (Fig. 180) thus only with auricular cartilage that grew normally, became delicate and flexible, and allowed a functional meatomyringoplasty to be performed. In contrast, the left side was reconstructed with costal cartilage that gradually hardened, did not grow, and progressed with little delicacy in shape and to the touch, as can be seen in the photographs.

This was my first case of bilateral microtia with auriculoplasty constructed exclusively with local microtial cartilage, attempting to show the expansion would work to obtain full size and a flexible ear. Scale designs (Fig. 181) show both pre- and postoperative height and width in millimeters to demonstrate the expansion. The conchal deficiency was corrected later with the canal construction.

Figure 180

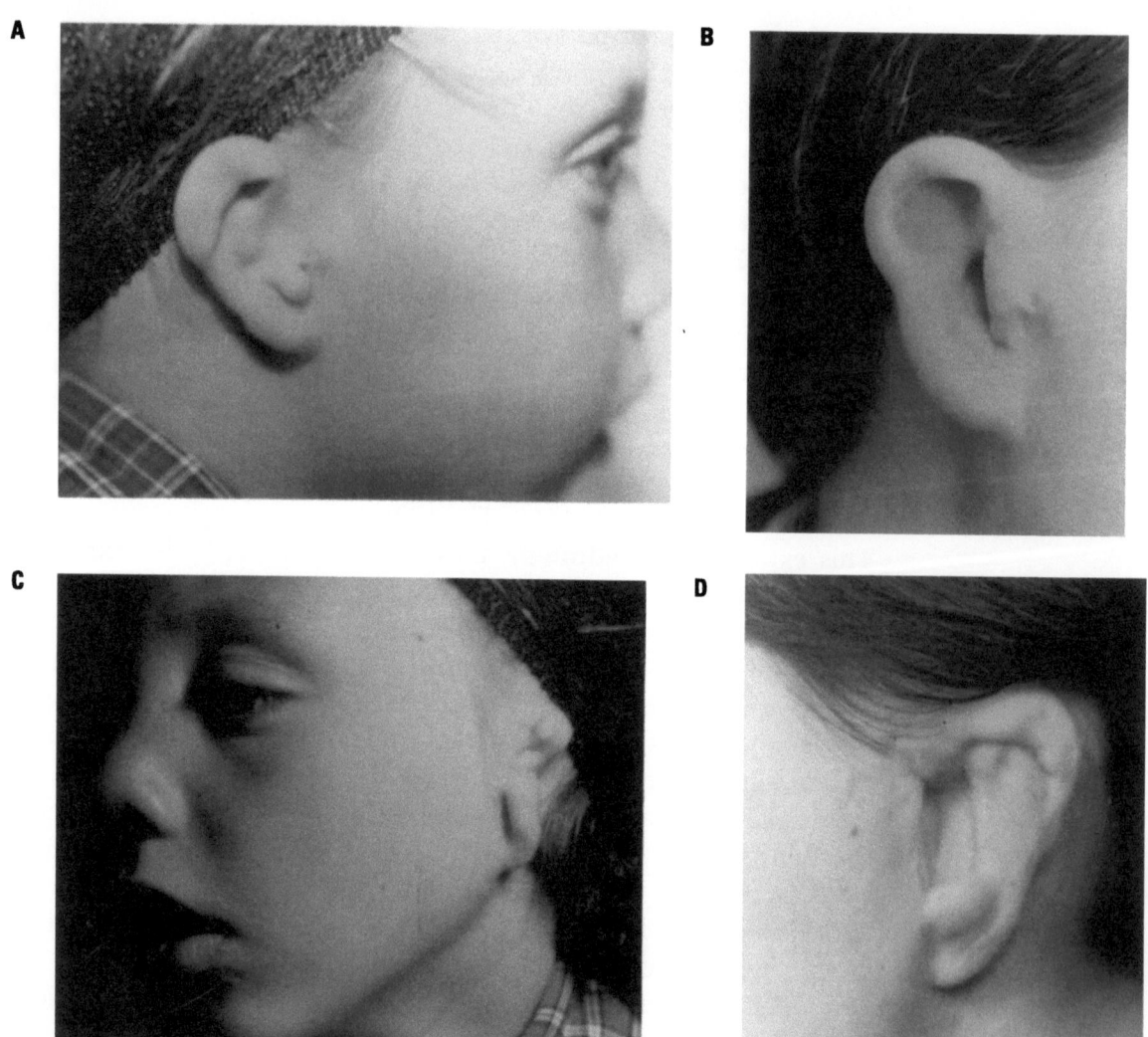

Figure 181

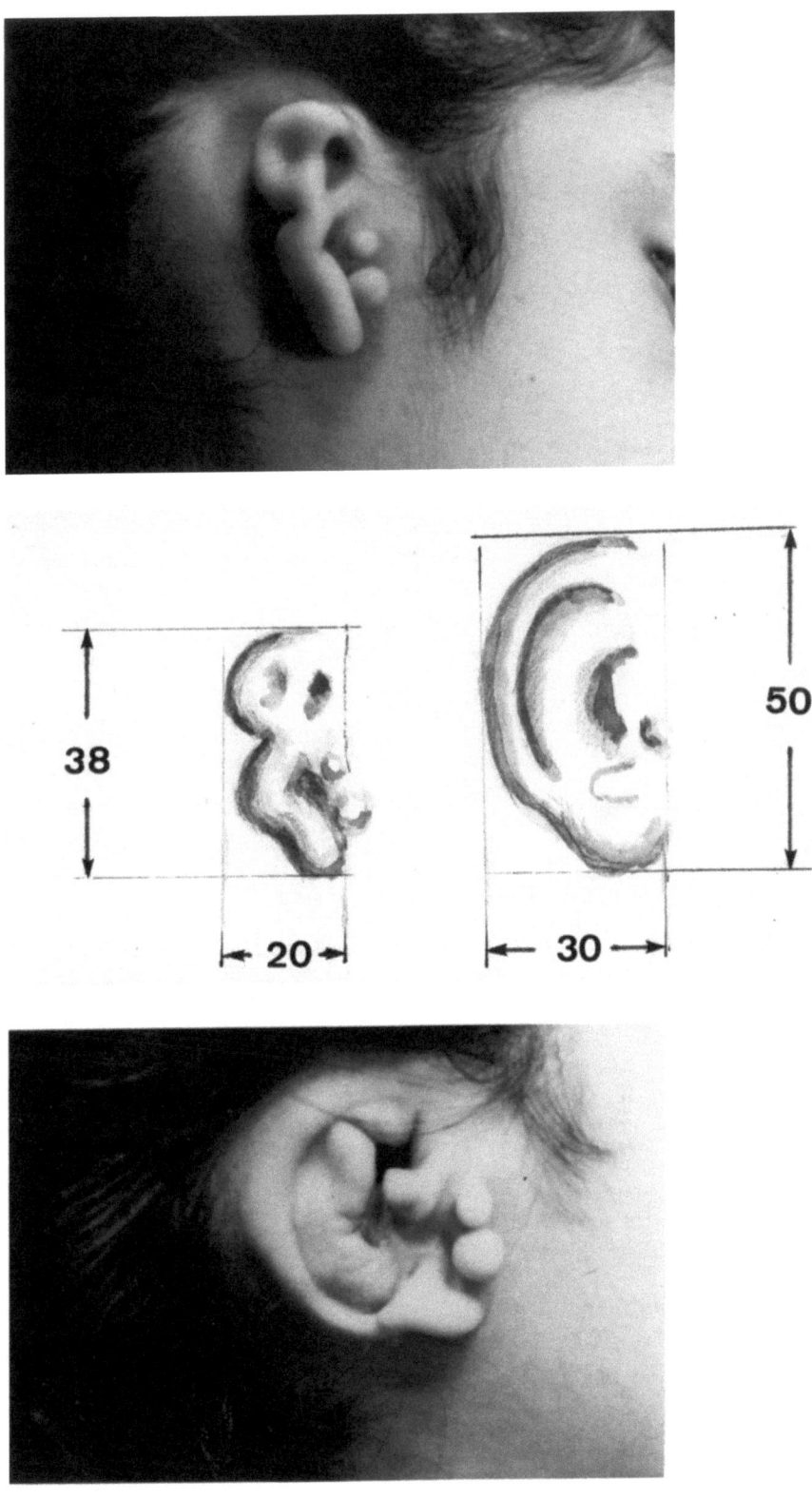

Severe Microtia Repaired Only with Microtial Cartilage of the Same Side

In our practice we have kept to our principles, including when treating severe bilateral microtia. Each experience is a step forward as shown by the following case. This 14-year-old boy with severe bilateral microtia and total atresia is an example of our current results. He had been operated on when

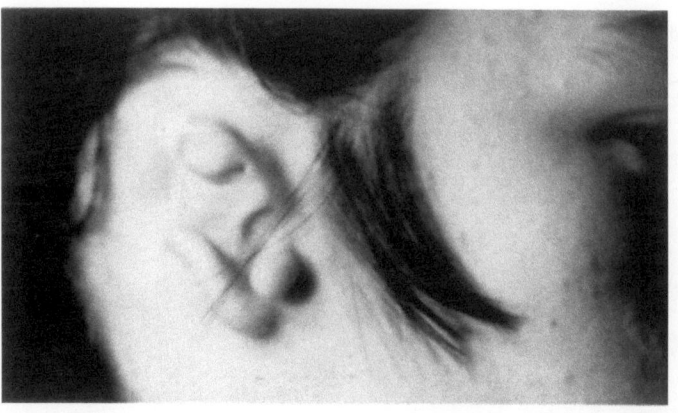 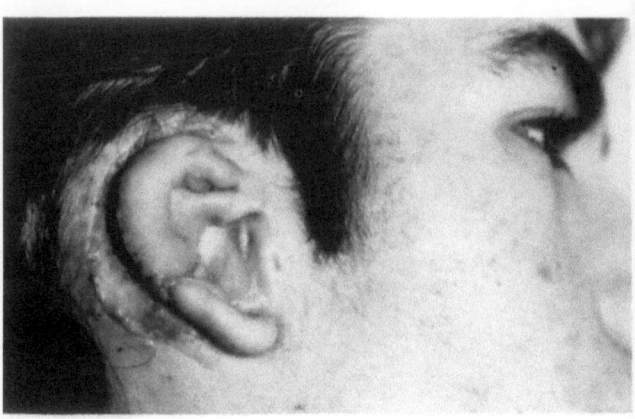

Figure 182
(A) The rib cartilage mass on the right side was reshaped with some improvement. (B) However, it remained fixed, rigid, hard, and obvious.

a boy at 6 years of age. Previous surgery had consisted of totally removing all vestiges of microtial cartilage, and implanting a poorly sculpted costal cartilage mass into the right aural area. The left side had remained untouched.

Repair commenced with exposure and reshaping of the costal cartilage on the right side, and then raising the ear with a retroaural skin graft. This served to measure the healing potential. Some improvement was obtained, but the ear remained firm, hard, gross, ugly, and without sensation (Fig. 182).

Later the left side was approached; it was virgin territory. The left microtia was classified as a severe "canoe" type, with total atresia. Reconstruction was with "bud that blooms" expansion chondroplasty, as previously described. The expansion has been designed and measured. The auricular result is illustrated (Fig. 183). The ear became normal in size, position, and to the touch. Mild, moderate, and maximum flexion and elasticity are shown (Fig. 184). Auriculoplasty had been performed in two stages, and upheld only with native cartilage (Fig. 185).

Figure 183
(Patient referred for surgery by Dr. Horacio García Igarza.)

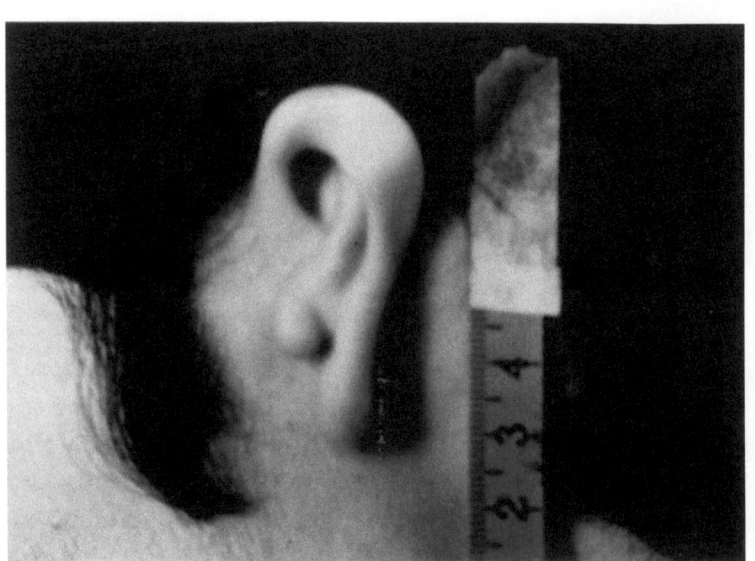 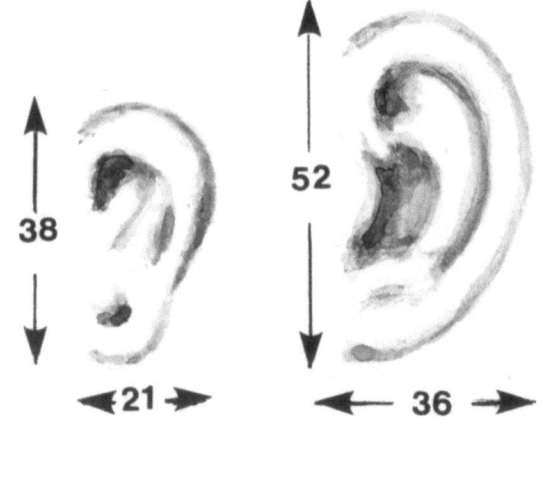

Chapter Six **Bilateral Microtia and Atresia**

Figure 184

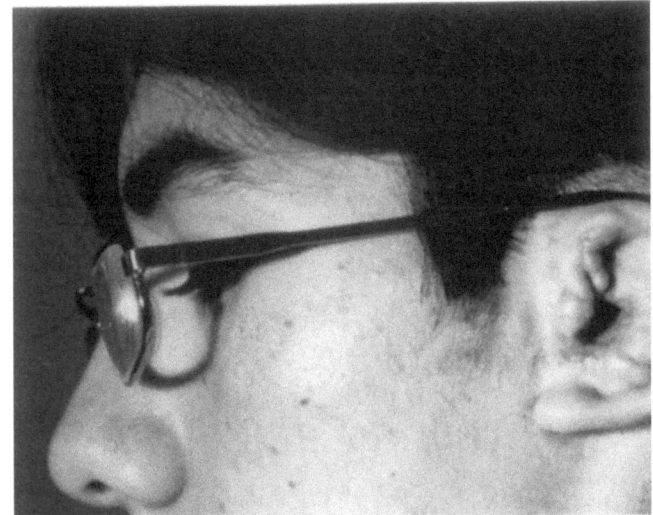

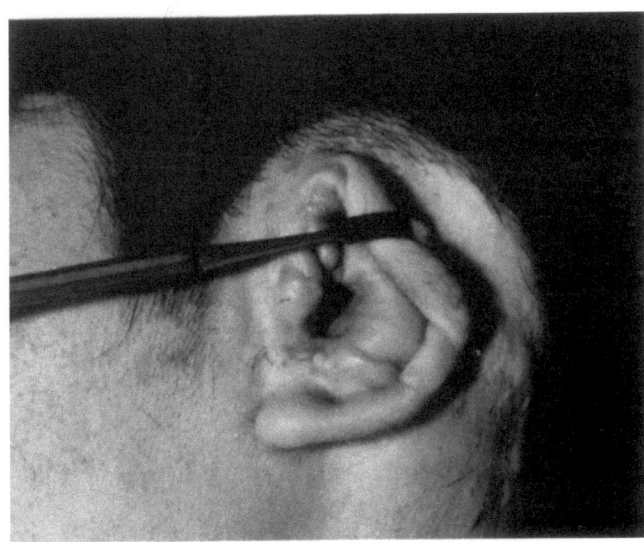

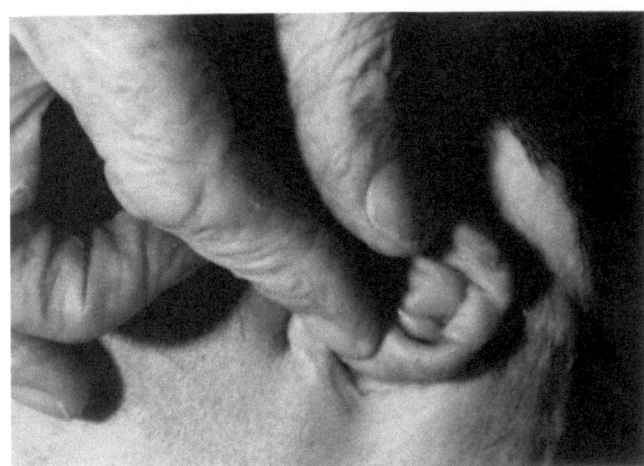

Severe Microtia Repaired Only with Microtial Cartilage of the Same Side

Figure 185

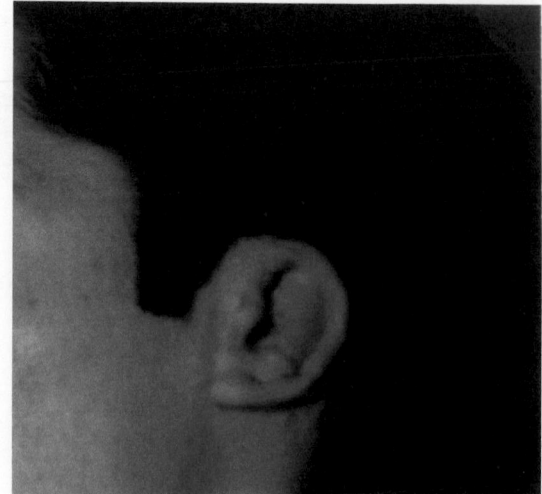

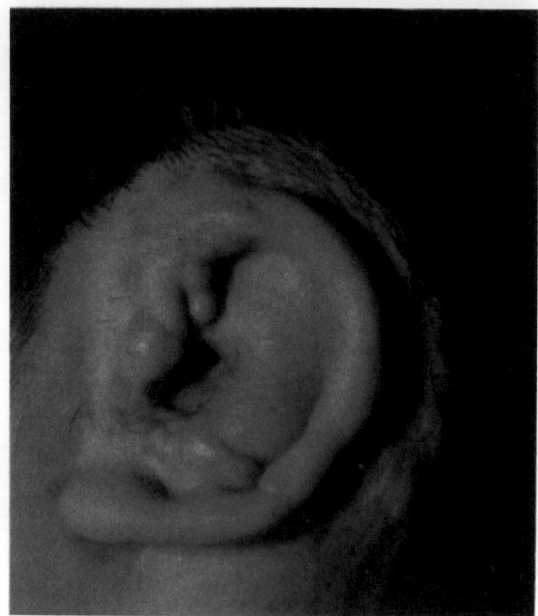

7
Hemifacial Microsomia

A house is enhanced by its garden. A jewel by its setting. And the ear by its surrounding tissues. They should be clear, clean, attractive, and unscarred.

Neighboring tissue is included in auriculoplasty. In the same manner that hairless skin is necessary to cover the helix, once the ear has been made, ample skin should be grafted into the retroaural sulcus to raise the organ. This bald graft is now discussed. It is well to reduce this bald area by replacing it with hairbearing or normal skin. The choice depends on hair density. Thick, dark hair is usually better that thin, transparent, blond hair. The graft area is reduced by the following methods:

1. Skin thickness cervical "lifting" flaps are brought up from below, and the lower visible graft border can easily be raised 30 mm.
2. Retroaural quadrangle scalp flaps are advanced forward. However, they do add needless scars and produce a hairline step deformity. Tanzer* has rotated a scalp flap downward.
3. The upper graft angle is usually obvious because it combines with the lack of a sideburn. There is also insufficient parotid development. These factors have been considered together to (a) fill the upper parotid depression, (b) construct the sideburn, and (c) camouflage the microsomia. This has been achieved with a rotation transposition full-thickness scalp flap taken from the temporomastoid area, switched forward into place and combined with the conchal scoop-out flap brought into the lower parotid area to fill it. Simultaneous chin repositioning balances the microsomia asymmetry in moderate cases.

The following case is of a young woman with a severe peanut microtia and total atresia (Fig. 186). Note the surrounding areas. There was no sideburn and no hair to camouflage the auricular deformity. There was a marked depression due to the absent parotid gland. The microsomia was obvious because the mandibular asymmetry (measured from the TM joint to mid-chin) was more than the tolerated difference of 10 mm (12 mm in this case).

The patient was corrected by stages. At the first, a temporal scalp flap was transposed forward to shape the sideburn and also fill in the upper

---

*Tanzer RC. An analysis of ear reconstruction. *Plast Reconstruct Surg.* 1963;31:16.

Figure 186

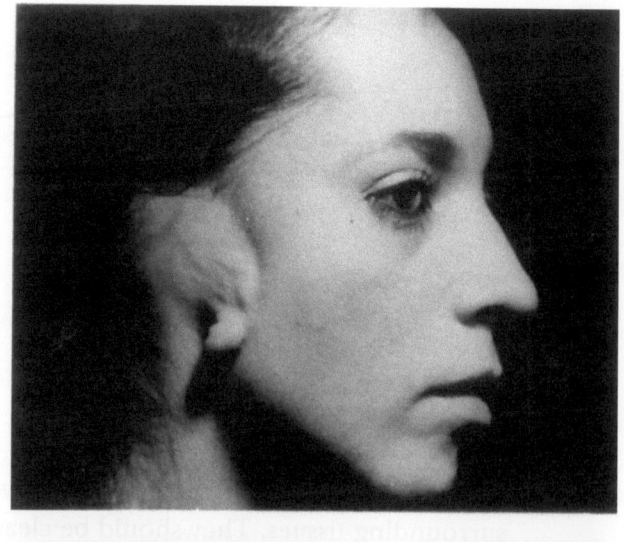

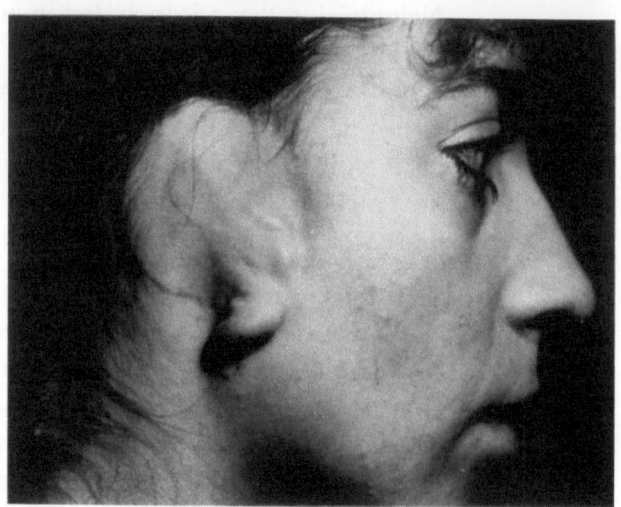

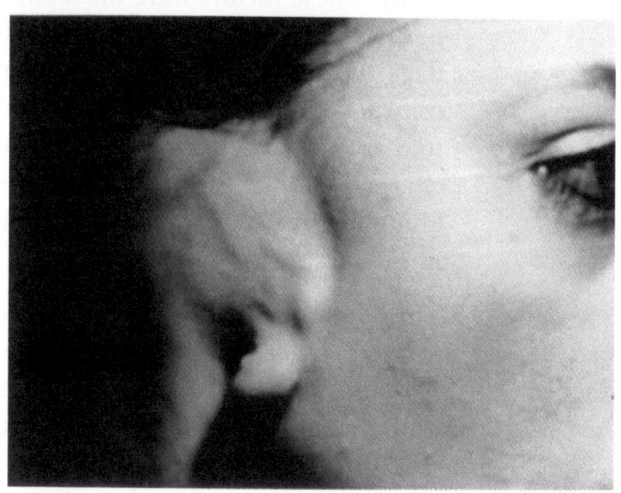

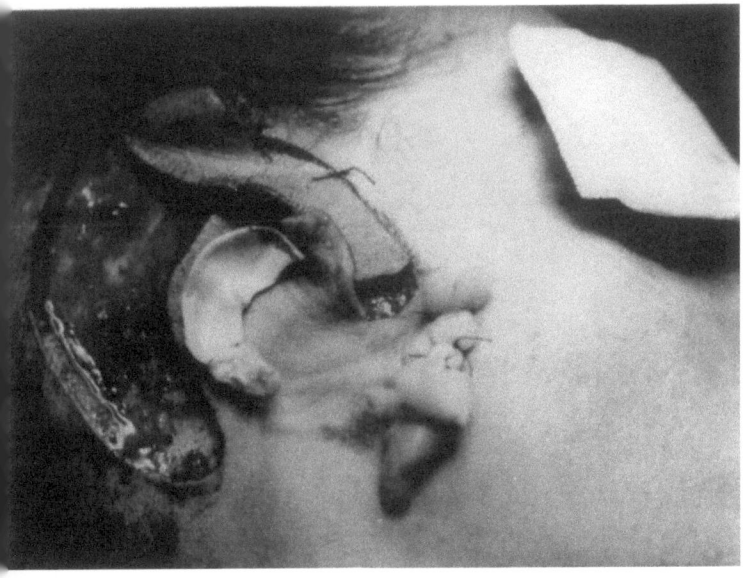
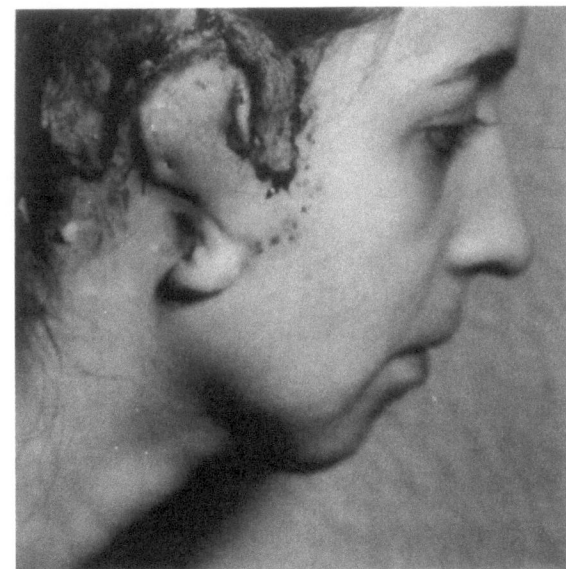

Figure 187

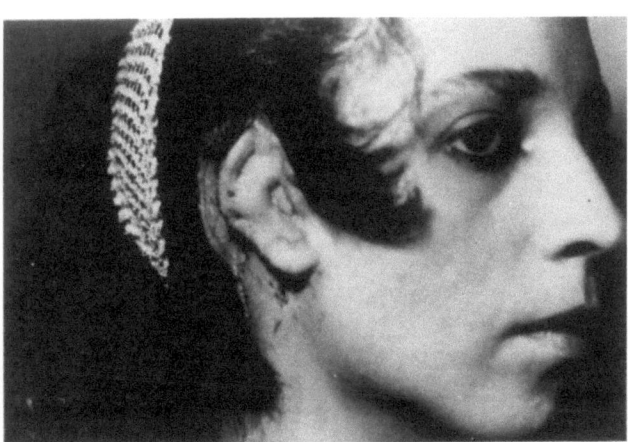
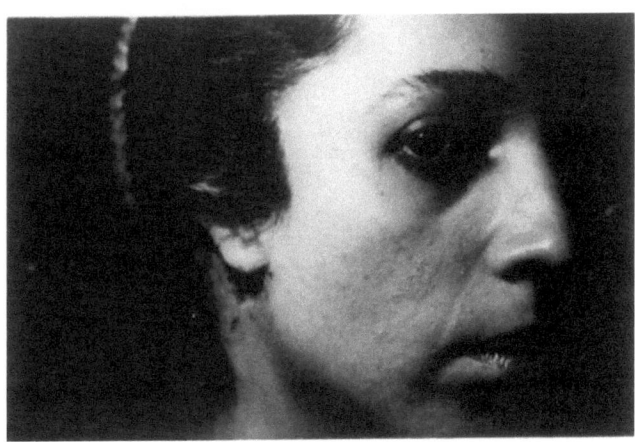

Figure 188

parotid depression. Simultaneously, contralateral conchal cartilage was brought in to form the upper auricle, and the concha was deepened. The conchal scooped-out tissue was rotated on the lower vascular pedicle, and used as a flap to fill in the lower parotid depression. The actual microtia was not touched (Fig. 187).

At the second stage the microtia was raised to connect with the helix, and the auricular sulcus deepened and skin-grafted, thus shaping the auricle (Fig. 188).

At the third stage meatomyringoplasty was performed. The microsomia was treated by bringing the deviated chin to the mid-line and taking a strip of the bony border from the larger side to pronounce the lesser, by grafting subperiostally (Fig. 189). The microtia, atresia, parotid depression, sideburns, and mandibular asymmetry were treated with these three operations over a period of 6 months.

Figure 189

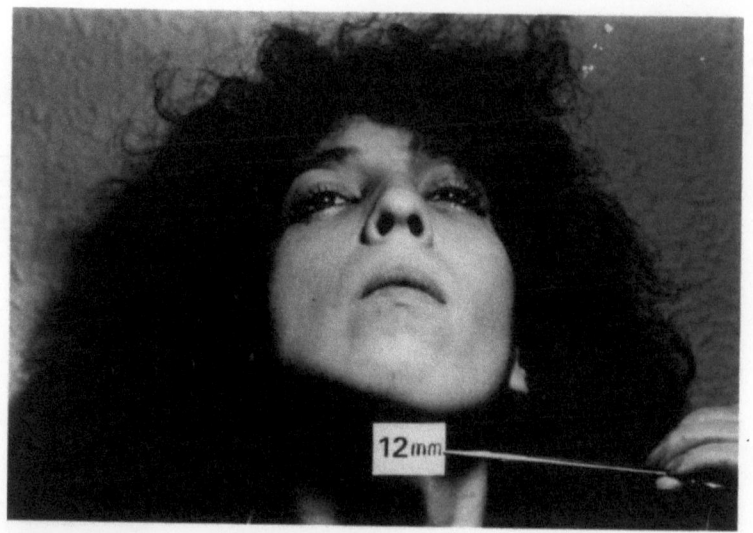

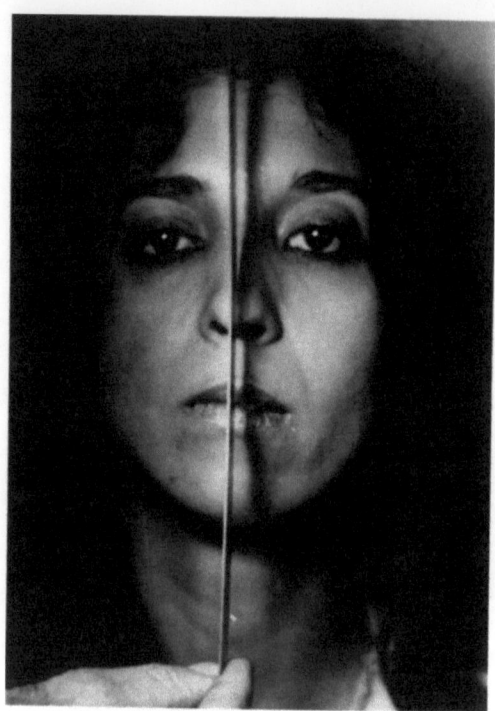

Measure of Results

Gillies classified a good result of radical ear repair when it was indistinguishable from the other side of a dark room. Peet stated that a good result was one that was not noticed by a passerby in the street. Tanzer claimed that a good result was when both the patient and the surgeon were satisfied.

At this stage, I consider that the measure of a satisfactory result is an organ that is within normal limits when seen and felt at an arm's length, can be flexed between the fingers, has extrinsic muscle movement, normal growth, and trophism, complies with full functional properties of an aural viscera, and has social hearing and stereognosis.

The goal is not only to make something that looks like an ear, but to create an organ that is an auricle; that is to say, perform not only auriculoplasty but functional auriculoplasty.

8 Conclusion

In 1959 Radford Tanzer[1] wrote, "One hesitates to generalize on a method buttressed by two completed cases. However, it seems fair to state that a technique of ear reconstruction has been devised which is applicable to several types of microtia, ... a firm knowledge of the principles involved in the manipulation of tissue with minimal scaring." He created history in ear repair.*

This book has contributed new solutions for a group of problems, as surgery has advanced. Applied new techniques, such as high-resolution computed tomography, magnetic resonance, high-resolution light microscopy, electronic microscopy, and microphotography, have contributed to better examinations, better diagnosis, and perfected surgery.

But the most important reevaluation has come with embryonic, functional, and chondral research, which has changed conceptions. Understanding microtia-atresia-microsomia to be one syndrome, and the principle of making the ear not only look human but also be human, has created a new outlook. Auricular cartilage framework, expansion chondrotomy, and otosurgery and plastic surgery teamwork form a new dimension, the value of which is not necessarily statistical. Attempting to analyze and establish a breakdown of my 92 completed ear reconstructions with rib cartilage and 352 with ear cartilage is rather pointless. There are too many variables for the results to be mathematically significant.

As each case is different, method selection depends on the patient's type of microtia and atresia and the surgeon's ability to use the native cartilage. Ear cartilage is the material of choice. The pre-endaural approach to the middle ear has proved to be the best. However, when anotic cartilage is reduced to a minimum in bilateral cases, there is no alternative but to use costal cartilage. This is the exception, not the rule. It is a poor standby to be used, realizing that the final outcome will not be the best.

On the horizon looms specialized cartilage culture, intrauterine microsurgery by cesarean section, and in situ endoscopy. As Longfellow wrote in "The Village Blacksmith," "Something attempted, something done, has earned a night's repose" (1840).

---

*Tanzer HC. Total reconstruction of the external ear. *Plast Reconstruct Surg.* 1959;23:1.

Bibliography*

Absi D, Trigo G, Buquet J, Sturla F. Osteotomía horizontal en escalón extendido a malar. Su aplicación en un caso de microsomía hemifacial. In: *XVII Congreso Argentino de Cirugía Plástica*, Resúmenes (abstracts). Buenos Aires: 1987.

Aguilar EA. A recent advance in auricular reconstruction. *Arch Otolaryngol Head Neck Surg.* 1991;117:1226.

Aguilar EA, Jahrsdoerfer RA. The surgical repair of congenital microtia and atresia. *Otolaryngol Head Neck Surg.* 1988;98:600.

Albrektsson T, Branemark PI, Jacobsson M, Tjellstöm A. Present clinical applications of osseointegrated percutaneous implants. *Plast Reconstr Surg.* 1987;79:721.

Alcaino AQ. Estudio embriológico, anatómico, etiológico, radiográfico, clínico y anatomo-quirúrgico de las agenesias del oido externo y medio. In: Remorino A, ed. *Actas del Primer Congreso Extraordinario de la Sociedad Internacional de Audiologia*. Buenos Aires: Guillermo Kraft; 1956:160.

Alexander G. Zur chirurgischen behandlung der kongenitalen atresie. *Z Ohrenh.* 1908;55:144.

Allison GR. Anatomy of the auricle. In: Furnas DW, ed. Reconstructive Surgery for Deformities of the Ear. *Clin Plast Surg.* 1990;17:209.

Allison GR, Achauer BM, Furnas DW. Growth of homotransplanted ear cartilage in baby rabbits. *Plast Reconstr Surg.* 1975;55:479.

Altman F. Congenital atresia of the ear in man and animals. *Ann Otol Rhinol Laryngol.* 1955;64:824.

Anitua M. Consideraciones embriológicas y anatomía quirúrgica de la cara. *Cir Plast Ibero-Lat Am.* 1976;2:17,63.

Anson BJ, Bast TH. The surgical significance of the stapedial and labyrinthine anatomy. *Q Bull Northwestein Univ Med School.* 1958;32:307.

Anson BJ, Donaldson JA. *Surgical Anatomy of the Temporal Bone.* Philadelphia: W.B. Saunders; 1981.

Apesos J, Kane M. Treatment of earlobe cleft. *Aesthetic Plast Surg.* 1993;17:253.

Argamaso RV. Ear reduction with or without setback otoplasty. *Plast Reconstr Surg.* 1989;83:967.

Argamaso RV. Ear reduction. Reply (correspondence). *Plast Reconstr Surg.* 1990;85:316.

Argamaso RV. An ideal site for auricular composite graft. *Br J Plast Surg.* 1975;28:219.

Argamaso RV. A simplified dressing for the earlobe. *Br Plast Surg.* 1977;30:100.

Argamaso RV, Lewin ML. The lateral transhelical approach for correction of deformities of the external ear. *Aesthetic Plast Surg.* 1978;2:157.

Argenta LC, Watanabe MJ, Grabb WC. The use of soft tissue expanders in head and neck reconstruction. *Ann Plast Surg.* 1983;11:31.

Ariyan S, Chicarilli Zeno N. Replantation of a totally amputated ear by means of a platysma musculo-cutaneous "sandwich" flap. *Plast Reconstr Surg.* 1986;78:385.

Attwood AI, Evans DM. Correction of prominent ears using Mustardés technique: an out-patient procedure under local anaesthetic in children and adults. *Br J Plast Surg.* 1985;38:252.

Aufricht G. The development of plastic surgery in the United States. *Plast Reconstr Surg.* 1946;7:3.

Aufricht G. Philosophy of cosmetic surgery. *Plast Reconstr Surg.* 1957;2:397.

Avakoff JC. A simple auricular chondrocutaneous flap. *Plast Reconstr Surg.* 1986;77:843.

---

*Davis J,E. *Aesthetic and Reconstructive Otoplasty*. New York; Springer-Verlag; 1987.

Avelar JM. Auriculo plastías en un solo tiempo. Presented in: *Argentine Society of Plastic Surgery Congress.* Argentina: Mendoza; 1990.

Avelar JM. Deformidades auriculares. In: Avelar JM, ed. *Cirurgia Plástica na Infância.* Sao Paulo: Editorial Hipócrates; 1989:279–384.

Avelar JM. *Cirurgia Plastica na Infância.* Sao Paulo: Cidade Editora Cientifica; 1989.

Avelar JM. Congenital deformities of the auricle. Experience of 138 cases of ear reconstruction. *Rev Soc Brasil Cir Plast.* 1986;1:28.

Avelar JM. Importance of ear reconstruction for the aesthetic balance of the facial contour. In: *Proceedings of the VIII ISAPS Congress.* Madrid: 1985:11.

Avelar JM. Importance of ear reconstruction for the aesthetic balance of the facial contour. *Aesthetic Plast Surg.* 1986;10:147.

Avelar JM. A personal approach to improve the results of ear reconstruction. In: Maneksha RJ, ed. *Transactions IX International Congress of Plastic and Reconstructive Surgery.* New Delhi, McGraw-Hill; 1987:557.

Avelar JM. Personal communication. 1990.

Avelar JM. Reconstrucão auricular primaria. In: Avelar, JM, ed. *Cirurgia Plastica na Infância.* Sao Paulo: Cidade Editora Cientifica; 1989:291.

Avelar JM. Retalho de fáscia creneana (galea). Anatomia, planejamento e aplição cirúgica. In: Avelar, JM, ed. *Cirurgia Plastica na Infância.* Sao Paulo: Cidade Editora Cientifica; 1989:314.

Avelar JM. Reconstrução do pólo superior da orelha. In: Avelar, JM, ed. *Cirurgia Plastica na Infancia.* Sao Paulo: Cidade Editora Cientifica; 1989:331.

Avelar JM. Reconstrução do lóbulo auricular. In: Avelar, JM, ed. *Cirurgia Plastica na Infância.* Sao Paulo: Cidade Editora Cientifica; 1989:338.

Avelar JM. Reconstrução auricula pós-traumática. In: Avelar, JM, ed. *Cirurgia Plastica na Infância.* Sao Paulo: Cidade Editora Cientifica; 1989:343.

Avelar JM. Reconstrução auricular pós-queimadura. In: Avelar, JM, ed. *Cirurgia Plastica na Infância.* Sao Paulo: Cidade Editora Cientifica; 1989:351.

Avelar JM. Reconstrução secundaria da orelha. In: Avelar, JM, ed. *Cirurgia Plastica na Infância.* Sao Paulo: Cidade Editora Cientifica; 1989:358.

Avelar JM. Complicações em reconstrução auricular. In: Avelar, JM, ed. *Cirurgia Plastica na Infância.* Sao Paulo: Cidade Editora Cientifrica; 1989:364.

Avelar JM, Bocchino F. Embriologia da orelha. In: Avelar, JM, ed. *Cirurgia Plastica na Infância.* Sao Paulo: Cidade Editora Cientifica; 1989:279.

Avelar JM, Bocchino F. Anatomia da orelha. In: Avelar, JM, ed. *Cirurgia Plastica na Infância.* Sao Paulo: Cidade Editora Cientifica; 1989:283.

Avelar JM, Malbec EF. Cirugía del pabellón auricular. In: Avelar, JM, Malbec, EF, eds. *Historia, Ciencia y Arte en Cirugía Estetica.* Sao Paulo: Editora Hipocrates; 1990:354,401–449.

Avelar JM, Psillakis JM. Microtia: total reconstruction of the auricle in one single operation. *Br J Plast Surg.* 1981;34:224.

Baker DC, Rees TD. Problems and complications in otoplasty. In: Lewis JR Jr., ed. *The Art of Aesthetic Plastic Surgery.* Boston: Little, Brown; 1989:305.

Bardsley AF. Ear salvage by the temporoparietal island flap. *Br J Plast Surg.* 1989;84:1010.

Bardsley AF. Primary reconstruction of a severed ear fragment using a flap of temporo-paretal fascia. *Br J Plast Surg.* 1986;39:524.

Bardsley AF, Mercer DM. The injured ear. A review of 50 cases. *Br J Plast Surg.* 1983;36:466.

Barinka L. Congenital and acquired auricular deformities: their reconstruction by a new technique. In. Robbett WF, ed. *Proceedings of the Centennial Symposium, Manhattan Eye, Ear, and Throat Hospital,* St. Louis: C.V. Mosby; 1969:187.

Barinka L. *Reconstruction of Auricle.* Brno: J.E. Purkyne University Press; 1987.

Barinka L. Reconstruction of Auricle (Rekonstrukee Boltce). Book review by Blair O. Rogers. *Aesthetic Plast Surg.* 1990;14:79.

Barragan F, Rodriguez H, Fuente F de la, Ceballo J, Prieto M. Quick and simple technique for the anatomical recontruction of the concha auriculae. *Aesthetic Plast Surg.* 1992;16:265.

Bast TH, Anson B. Timetable of development of the ear. In: Coates, GM, ed. *Otorhinolaringology.* Hagerstown, W.F. Prior; 1955.

Baudet J. Successful replantation of a large severed ear fragment. *Plast Reconstr Surg.* 1973;51:82.

Bauer BS. Reconstruction of the microtic ear. *J Pediatr Surg.* 1984;19:440.

Bauer BS. The role of tissue expansion in reconstruction of the ear. Furnas, DW, ed. In: Reconstructive Surgery for Deformities of the Ear. *Clin Plast Surg.* 1990;17:319.

Beers MD. Surgical management of the auricular lobule. In: Masters, FW, Lewis, JR, eds. *Symposium on Aesthetic Surgery of the Nose, Ears, and Chin.* St. Louis: C.V. Mosby; 1973:165.

Beker OJ. Surgical correction of the abnormally protruding ear. *Arch Otolaryngol.* 1959;50:541.

Bellucci RJ. Congenital aural malformations: diagnosis and treatment. *Otolaryngol Clin North Am.* 1981;14:95.

Bellucci RJ. The problem of congenital auricular malformations. *Trans Am Acad Ophtalmol Otolaryngol.* 1960;64:840.

Benmeir P, Neuman A, Weinberg A, Wexler MR. Team approach to total auricular reconstruction. *Ann Plast Surg.* 1992;28:397.

Bennum RD, Mulliken JB, Kaban LB, Murray JE. Microtia: a microform of hemifacial microsomia. *Plast Reconstr Surg.* 1985;76:859.

Berger JC. An unusual case of keloidal scars of the ears. *Plast Reconstr Surg.* 1955;16:474.

Berhaus A, Toplak F. Surgical concept for reconstruction of auricle: history and current status of the art. *Arch Otolaryngol Head Neck Surg.* 1986;112:388.

Berthold E. Ueber myringoplastik. *Wien Med Bl.* 1878;1:627.

Bezanzon C. Les otopoièses dans les malformations de l'oreille externe. *Thèse Méd Nancy.* 1980;283.

Blake CJ. Middle ear operations. *Trans Am Otol Soc.* 1892;5:306.

Bochnia M, Ziemski Z, Dus E, Lesniakowska E. Several generations of developmental abnormalities of the branchial arches cleft. *Otolaryngol Pol.* 1992;46:80.

Boles RC, Teebi AS, Schwartz D, Harper JF. Further delineation of the ear patella, short stature syndrome (Meir-Gorlin syndrome). *Clin Dysmorphol.* 1994;3:207.

Boo-Chai K. The pixie earlobe: a method of correction. *Plast Reconstr Surg.* 1985;76:636.

Botta SA. A technique for otoplasty. *Aesthethic Plast Surg.* 1991;15:339.

Boucheron E. La movilisation de l'étrier et son procédé operatoire. *Union Méd Paris.* 1888;46:412.

Boudard P. Les techniques chirurgicales de reconstruction du pavillon de l'oreille dans les agénèsis majeures: mise au point d'un protocole therapeutique. *Thèse Med Bordeaux.* 1985;333.

Boudard P, Portmann M. Technique chirugicale de reconstruction totale du pavillon de l'oreille dans le case de agénésie majeure: utilisation d'un greffon cartilagineux costal. *Rev Laryngol.* 1987;108:507.

Brent, B. Auricular repair with autogenous rib cartilage grafts: two decades of experience with 600 cases. *Plast Reconstr Surg.* 1992;90:355.

Brent B. Reconstruction of the auricle. In: *Plastic Surgery.* Philadelphia: W.B. Saunders; 1990:2094.

Brent B. Reconstruction of ear. In: Grabb WC, Smith JW, eds. *Plastic Surgery: A Concise Guide to Clinical Practice.* Boston: Little, Brown; 1979.

Brent, B. The versatile cartilage autograft: current trends in clinical transplantation. *Clin Plast Surg.* 1979; 6:163.

Brent, B. *The Artistry of Reconstructive Surgery.* Brent B, Brent BP, eds. St. Louis: C.V. Mosby; 1987.

Brent, B. Auricular repair with a conchal cartilage graft. In: Brent B, Brent BP, eds. *The Artistry of Reconstructive Surgery.* St. Louis, C.V. Mosby; 1987:107.

Brent, B. Total auricular construction with sculpted costal cartilage. In: Brent B, Brent BP, eds. *The Artistry of Reconstructive Surgery.* St. Louis: C.V. Mosby; 1987:113.

Brent, B. Auricular construction with a fascial transposition flap. In: Brent B, Brent BP, eds. *The Artistry of Reconstructive Surgery.* St. Louis: C.V. Mosby; 1987:129.

Brent, B. Personal communication. 1988.

Brent, B, Finseth F. Microsurgical ear and scalp reconstruction with a fascia-cutaneous free flap. In: Brent B, Brent BP, eds. *The Artistry of Reconstructive Surgery.* St. Louis: C.V. Mosby; 1987:139.

Brent B, Upton J, Acland RD, et al. Experience with the temporoparietal fascial free flap. *Plast Reconstr Surg.* 1985;76:177.

Buchele BA, Zook EG. Altered spatial perception following harvest of a posterior auricular skin graft. *Plast Reconstr Surg.* 1988;81:954.

Buncke HJ. Microsurgical reattachment of totally amputated ears. Discussion. *Plast Reconstr Surg.* 1987;79:541.

Butler LC. Correction of the unilateral lop ear. Presented at the *Texas Society for Plastic Surgery.* Dallas, April 27, 1963.

Byars LT, Anderson R. Anomalies of the first branchial cleft. *Surg Gynecol Obstet.* 1951;93:755.

Cabral LM. Oreja prominente: desarrollo de la técnica de dos vías. In: *I Congreso Uruguayo de Cirugía Plástica, XXIV Jornadas Rioplatenses del Cono Sud.* Punta del Este: 1987.

Caldarelli DD, Hutchinson JC, Pruzansky S, Valvassori G. Hemifacial microsomia: priorities and sequence of comprehensive therapy. In: *Third International Congress on Cleft Palate and Related Craneofacial Anomalies.* Abstracts. Toronto: 1977.

Caldarelli DD, Hutchinson JC, Pruzansky S, Valvassori GE. A comparison of microtia and temporal bone anomalies in hemifacial microsomia and mandibulofacial dysostosis. *Cleft Palate.* 1980;17:103.

Campbell G. Otoplasty: something old, something new. Reconstruction of the external ear using fresh cadaver homograft ear cartilage and a sternomastoid myocutaneous flap. *Br J Plast Surg.* 1983;36:262.

Candas O. Personal communications.

Candas OE, Davis JE, Martinez M. Investigación mediante tomografia computada del abordaje del oido medio en las microtias. Presented at the *XXII*

Panamerican Congress of Otorhinolaryngology, Head and Neck Surgery, Buenos Aires, December 1990.

Cannon B. New honors for Joseph E. Murray and Radford C. Tanzer. *Plast Reconstr Surg.* 1987;80:753.

Cano I, Encinas A, Herrero E, Lagaron E, Villarino A, Berchi FJ. The indications, technics and results of the use of tissue expanders in pediatric surgery. *Circ Pediatr.* 1991;4:173.

Cano I, Encinas A, Herrero E, Lagaron E, Villarino A, Berchi FJ. The indications, technics and results of the use of tissue expanders in pediatric surgery, *Cir. Pediatr.* 1991;4:173.

Caputo V, Cansiglio V. The use of patient's own auricular cartilage to repair deficiency of the tracheal wall. *J Thorac Cardiovasc Surg.* 1961;41:594.

Carey JS. Called as an expert witness. *Br Med J.* 1986;293:1658.

Castilla EE, Orioli IM. Prevalence rates of microtia in South America. *Int J Epidemiol.* 1986;15:364.

Celsus, quoted by Heine B, Beck J. In: Denker A, Kahler O, eds. *Handbuch der Hals-nasen-oherenheilknunde*, vol. 8. Berlin: 1927.

Chang YL, Chen YR, Noordhoff MS. Reconstruction of the middle third auricular defect based on aesthetic perception theory. *Aesthetic Plast Surg.* 1990;14:223.

Chavoin JP, Ruaux C, Rouge D, Fradin N, Costagliola M. Otoplasties pour oreilles décollées. *Ann Chir Plast Esthet.* 1990;35:303.

Chen ZJ. *Abstracts of papers presented at the First National Conference of Burn and Plastic Surgery*. Beijing: Chinese Medical Association; 1982:128.

Chen ZJ. One stage total auricle reconstruction and reestablishment of hearing in severe congenital microtia. *Ann Chir Plast Esthet.* 1988;33:335.

Chin DTW, Chen L, Chen ZW. Rat ear reattachment as an animal model. *Plast Reconstr Surg.* 1990;85:782.

Clark RP. Ear reduction. *Plast Reconstr Surg.* 1990;85:316.

Coccaro FJ, Becker MH, Converse JE. Clinical and radiographic variations in hemifacial microsomia. *Birth Defects.* 1975;2:314.

Coe HE. Correction of lop ears. *Northwest Med.* 1942;41:126.

Cohen B, Temple IK, Symons JC, et al. Microtia and short stature: a new syndrome. *J Med Genet.* 1991;28:786.

Cohen MM. Variability versus "incidental findings" in the first and second arch syndrome: unilateral variants with anophthalmia. *Birth Defects.* 1971;7:103.

Cole RR, Jahrsdoerfer RA. Congenital aural atresia. In: Furnas DW, ed. *Reconstructive Surgery for Deformities of the Ear. Clin Plast Surg.* 1990;17:367.

Colman BH. Congenital atresia: aspects of surgical care. *Acta Otorhinolaryngol Belg.* 1971;25:929.

Conley JJ, Novock AJ. The surgical removal of malignant tumors of the ear and temporal bone. *Arch Otorhinolaryngol.* 1960;71:635.

Conroy WC. Salvage of amputated ear. *Plast Reconstr Surg.* 1972;49:564.

Converse JM, McCarthy JG, Wood-Smith D. In: *Symposium on Diagnosis and Treatment of Craniofacial Anomalies.* St. Louis: C.V. Mosby; 1979.

Converse JM, Nicro A, Wilson FA, Johnson N. A technique for surgical correction of lop ears. *Trans Am Acad Ophtalmo Otolaryngol.* 1956;59:551.

Converse JM, Wood-Smith D, Coccaro PJ, Becker M. Bilateral facial microsomia. Diagnosis, classification and treatment. *Plast Reconstr Surg.* 1974;54:413.

Conway H, Howell JA. Carcinoma of the external ear. *Plast Reconstr Surg.* 1957;20:45.

Corey JP, Caldarelli OD, Gould HJ. Otopathology in cranial, facial disostosis. *Am J Otol.* 1987;8:14.

Cosman B. Repair of the constricted ear. In: Brent B, Brent BP, eds. *The artistry of reconstructive surgery.* St. Louis: C.V. Mosby; 1987:99.

Cotin G, Garabedian N, Lacombe H. Procédés de reconstruction du conduit auditif externe et du méat dans les aplasies de l'oreille et les sténoses. *Ann Chir Plast.* 1985;30:363.

Courtiss EH. An otoplasty technique. Lewis JR, Jr, ed. In: *The Art of Aesthetic Plastic Surgery.* Boston: Little, Brown; 1989:289.

Crane JP, Beaver HA. Midtrimester sonographic diagnosis of mandibulofacial dysostosis. *Am J Med Genet.* 1986;25:251.

Cremers WR, Smeets JH. Acquired atresia of the external auditory canal. Surgical treatment and result. *Arch Otolaryngol Head Neck Surg.* 1993;119:162.

Crestinu JM. The pretragal flap. *Br J Plast Surg.* 1981;34:295.

Daroda M. Utilización de colgajos de facia temporal para reconstrucción auricular. Presented at the *XX Congreso Argentino de Cirugía Plástica*, Mendoza, Argentina, 1990.

D'assumpçao EA. Corrección de orejas en abano con escarificación anterior del cartilago conchal. Presented at the I Congreso Uruguayo de Cirugía Plástica, *XXIV Jornadas Rioplatenses. II Jornadas del Cono Sud*, Punta del Este, 1987.

David DJ, Mahatumarat C, Cooter RD. Hemifacial microsomia: a multisystem classification. *Plast Reconstr Surg.* 1987;80:525.

David JB, Kitlowsky EA. Abnormal prominence of the ears: a method of readjustment. *Surgery.* 1937;2:835.

Davis JE. Prominent ears. In: Gonzales-Ulloa M, Meyer R, Smith JW, Zaoli G, eds. *Aesthetic Plastic Surgery*. Padova: Piccin Nuova Libraria; 1987:II:299.

Davis JE. Anatomy of the ear. In: Stark RB, ed. *Plastic Surgery of the Head and Neck*. New York: Churchill Livingstone; 1987:455.

Davis JE. Auriculoplastías. Presented at the *XVII Congreso Argentino de Cirugía Plástica*. Temas Centrales, abstracts, Buenos Aires, 1–4 Sept., 1987.

Davis, JE. *Aesthetic and Reconstructive Otoplasty*. New York: Springer-Verlag: 1987.

Davis JE. Aesthetic and reconstructive otoplasty. *Plast Reconstr Surg*. 1988;82:1095.

Davis JE. Aesthetic otoplasty. In: Lewis JR Jr, ed. *The Art of Aesthetic Plastic Surgery*. Boston: Little, Brown; 1989:265.

Davis JE. Conchal transposition flap for postburn ear deformities. Discussion. *Plast Reconstr. Surg*. 1989;83:653.

Davis JE. Auriculoplastia secundaria. Presented in: *Course of XX Congreso Argentino de Cirugía Plástica*. Mendoza, Argentina, 1990.

Davis JE. Auriculoplasty. Presented in: Course of *XX Congreso Argentino de Cirugía Plástica*. Mendoza, Argentina, 1990.

Davis JE. Auriculoplastías en el contexto de los 1. y 2. arcos branquiales. Presented at the Course of *XX Congreso Argentino de Cirugía Plástica*. Mendoza, Argentina, 1990.

Davis, JE. Auriculoplasty. Presented at the *XXVII Congresso Brasileiro de Chirurgia Plástica*. Rio de Janeiro, Brazil, 1990.

Davis JE. Cryptotia. Presented at the *International Society for Aesthetic Plastic Surgery Congress*. Jalisco, Mexico, 1992.

Davis JE, Cianflone, J. Otoplastias. Orejas prominentes. In: *Texto de Cirugía Plástica, Reconstructiva y Estética*. Coiffman F, ed. Barcelona: Salvat; 1986:823.

Davis JE, Cianflone J. Prominent ears. In: Ulloa MG, Meyer R, Smith J, Zaoli G, eds. *Aesthetic Plastic Surgery*. Piccin Nuova Libraria; 1987:299.

Davis JE, Hernandez HH. History of the aesthetic surgery of the ear. In: Gonzalez-Ulloa M, ed. *The Creation of Aesthetic Plastic Surgery*. New York: Springer-Verlag; 1985.

Davis PKB. An operation for hematoma auris. *Br J Plast Surg*. 1971;24:277.

Dean LW, Gittins TR. Report of a case of bilateral congenital osseous, atresia of the external auditory canal with exceptionally good functional result following operation. *Trans Am Laryngol Rhinol Otol Soc*. 1917.

Decourtioux JL. Un procede simple de correction chirurgicale de l'abscence congenitale de l'helix. *Ann Chir Plast*. 1971;16:60.

De La Fuente A, Casado C, Barron J, Pena MC. Colgajo libre dermograso para el tratamiento de la microsomia hemifacial. *Cir Plast Ibero-Lat Am*. 1980;6:67.

Dellon AL, Claybaugh GJ, Hoopes JE. Hemipalatal palsy and microtia. *Ann Plast Surg*. 1983;10:475.

Derlacki EL. Repair of central performations of tympanic membrane. *Arch Otolaryngol*. 1953;58:405.

Derlacki EL, Clemís JD. Congenital cholesteatoma of the middle ear and mastoid. *Ann Otol Rhinol Laryngol*. 1965;74:706.

De Isasa Gonzalez De Ubieta C. La oreja en la cultura. *Cir Plast Ibero-Lat Am*. 1990;16:71.

De Silva ED. Preaxial polidactyly and other defects associated with Klipper-Fell anomaly. *Hum Hered*. 1993;43:371.

Diamante VG. Personal communication.

Disant F, Lemblond J. Reconstruction of the external ear. *Rev Prat*. 1992;42:2069.

Diz Dios P, Garcia A, Fernandez Feijoo J, Castro Ferreira M, Alvarez FJ, Varela Otero J. An implant supported auricular prosthesis. *Acta Otorhinolaringol Esp*. 1994;45:45.

Donelan MB. Conchal transposition flap for postburn ear deformities. *Plast Reconstr Surg*. 1989;83:641.

Duato F, Moreno F, Cimorra G. Sindrome de Goldenhar. *Cir Plast Ibero-Lat Am*. 1977;3:153.

Dubs R. A new method for attaching an auricle prosthesis. *Pract Oto-rhinolaryngol*. 1965;27:172.

Dunham ME, Friedman HI. Audiologic management of bilateral external auditory canal atresia with bone conducting implantable hearing devise. *Cleft Palate J*. 1990;27:369.

Dupertuis SM. Free ear lobe grafts of skin and fat; their value in reconstruction about the nostril. *Plast Reconstr Surg*. 1946;1:135.

Eavey RD. Microtia and significant auricular malformation. Ninety two pediatric patients. *Arch Otolaryngol Head Neck Surg*. 1995;121:57.

Eavey RD. Personal communication, 1993.

Edgerton MT, Marsh JL. Surgical treatment of hemifacial microsomia (first and second branchial arch syndrome). *Plast Reconstr Surg*. 1977;59:653.

Eisemann ML. The growth potential of autograph cartilage. *Arch Otolaryngol*. 1983;109:469.

Elliott RA. Aesthetic surgery of the ears. In: Georgiade NG, Georgiade GS, Riefkohl R, Barwick WJ, eds. *Essentials of Plastic, Maxillofacial, and Reconstructive Surgery*. Baltimore: Williams and Wilkins; 1987:621.

Elliott RA. Developmental defects of the ear. Composite

otoplasty. In: Stark RB, ed. *Plastic Surgery of the Head and Neck*. New York: Churchill Livingstone; 1987:479.

Elliott RA. Otoplasty. In: Regnault P, Daniel RK, eds. *Aesthetic Plastic Surgery*. Boston: Little, Brown; 1984.

Elliott RA. Otoplasty: a combined approach. In: Furnas DW, ed. *Reconstructive Surgery for Deformities of the Ear. Clin Plast Surg*. 1990;17:373.

Elliott RA. Otoplasty for prominent ears. Composite otoplasty. In: Stark RB, ed. *Plastic Surgery of the Head and Neck*. New York: Churchill Livingstone; 1987:479.

Ellwood LC, Winter ST, Dar H. Familiar microtia with meatal atresia in two siblings. *J Med Genet*. 1968;5:289.

Elsahy NI. Reconstruction of the cleft earlobe with preservation of the perforation for an earring. *Plast Reconstr Surg*. 1986;77:322.

Elsahy NI. Technique for correction of lop ear. *Plast Reconstr Surg*. 1990;85:615.

Ely E. A classic reprint: an operation for prominence of the auricles. *Plast Reconstr Surg*. 1988;82:562.

Ely ET. A classic reprint: an operation for prominence of the auricles (with two wood-cuts). *Aesthetic Plast Surg*. 1987;11:73.

Eppley BL, Sadove AM. An improved draping method for otoplastic surgery. *Aesthetic Plast Surg*. 1990;14:293.

Escudeiro LH, Oliveira de Castro A. Reconstrução do canal auditivo nas malformações congénitas do aparello auditivo. In: Avelar JM, ed. *Cirugia plástica na infância*. Sao Paulo: Cidade Editora Cientifica; 1989:368.

Farkas LG. Anthropometry of the normal and defective ear. In: Furnas DW, ed. *Reconstructive Surgery for Deformities of the Ear. Clin Plast Surg*. 1990;17:213.

Fatah MF. L-plasty technique in the repair of split ear lobe. *Br J Plast Surg*. 1985;38:410.

Feuerstein SS, Adams JB. Surgery of the protruding ear. Course 1333. *Otolaryngol Head Neck Surg*. 1987;96:423.

Filippi NI. Hemifacial microsomia with vertebral anomalies: case report. *Birth Defects*. 1971;7:197.

Firmin F. Microtia. Reconstruction by Brent's technique. *Ann Chir Plast Esthet*. 1992;37:19.

Firmin F. Personal communication, 1991.

Firmin F, Raphaël B. Reconstruction du pavillon auriculaire. In: *Rapport du XXXIII Congrès de la Société Française de Chirurgie Plastique, Reconstructrice et Esthétique*. Paris: Editions R. Sicard; 1988.

Fonseca Ely J. Defeitos congenitos da face. Defeitos congenitos das orelhas. In: Fonseca ES, ed. *Chirurgia Plástica*. Río de Janeiro: Editora Guanabara Koogan S.A.; 1980:334.

Fonseca EJ. Small incision otoplasty for prominent ears. *Aesthetic Plast Surg*. 1988;12:63.

Fonseca EJ, Granemann AS, Pereira OJ. Orelha em abano (Revisâo de 100 casos). Presented at the *XXVII Congresso Brasileiro de Cirurgia Plástica*. Río de Janeiro, Brasil, 1990.

Foster CA, Sherman JE. External ear malformations. In: Stark RB, ed. *Plastic Surgery of the Head and Neck*. New York: Churchill Livingstone; 1987:485.

Francesconi G, Grassi C, Fenili O, Chiocchetti C. La nostra esperienza nel trattamento chirurgi dell'orecchio ad ansa. *Acta Otorhinolaryngol Ital*. 1982;2:163.

Freeman BS. Post tragal incision. *Plast Reconstr Surg*. 1987;80:147.

Friede L, Pandolfi P. Otoplastica secondo Mustardé; valutazione dei resultati a distanza. *Riv Ital Chir Plast*. 1983;15:54.

Friedmann I. Epidermoid cholesteatoma and cholesterol granuloma. *Ann Otol Rhinol Laryngol*. 1959;68:57.

Frühwald V. *Korrektive Chirurgie der Nase, Ohren und des Gesichtes*, 2nd ed. Vienna: Verlag Wilhem Maudrich; 1952:79.

Fry HJH. Cartilage and cartilage grafts. *Plast Reconstr Surg*. 1967;40:426.

Fuente GG, Microtia: ¿deformidad aislada o sindrome? Presented at the *International Society of Aesthetic Plastic Surgery Meeting and Iberolatinamerican Society of Plastic Surgery Congress*, for resident's award. Guadalajara, Mexico, 1978.

Fukuda O. Complications and postoperative problems in reconstruction of the microtic ear. In: Manesha RJ, ed. *Transactions of the IX International Congress of Plastic and Reconstructive Surgery*. New Delhi: McGraw-Hill; 1987:557.

Fukuda O. Long-term evaluation of modified Tanzer ear reconstruction. In: Furnas DW, ed. Reconstructive Surgery for Deformities of the Ear. *Clin Plast Surg*. 1990;17:241.

Fukuda O. Reconstruction of microtia with a contour-accentuated framework and supplemental coverage (by Hiroyasu Naka). Discussion. *Plast Reconstr Surg*. 1986;78:609.

Furnas DW. Correction of prominent ears with multiple sutures. In: Lewis JR, ed. *The Art of Aesthetic Plastic Surgery*. Boston: Little, Brown; 1989:279.

Furnas DW. Complications of surgery of the external ear. In: Furnas DW, ed. Reconstructive Surgery for Deformities of the Ear. *Clin Plast Surg*. 1990;17:305.

Furukawa H, Fukuda O, Yamada A, Harii K, Oda M, Murakami Y. Three cases of microtia with congenital cholesteatoma. *Jpn J Plast Reconstr Surg.* 1983;26:117.

Furukawa M, Mizutani Z, Hamada T. A simple operative procedure for the treatment of Stahl's ear. *Br J Plast Surg.* 1985;38:544.

Gasperoni C. Ear deformity: reconstruction of the ear lobe and the scarcity of skin (Italian). *Riv Ital Chir Plast.* 1983;15:67.

Gellis SS, Feingold M. Hemifacial microtia. *Am J Dis Child.* 1971;122:57.

Gershoni BR, Mandel H, Miller B, Sujov P, Braun J. Walker-Warburg syndrome with microtia and absent auditory canals. *Am J Med Genet.* 1990;37:87.

Gibson T. Flagellation and free grafting (case recorded by H. Dutrochet). *Br J Plast Surg.* 1961;8:195.

Gibson T, Davis WB. The fate of preserved bovine cartilage implants in man. *Br J Plast Surg.* 1953;6:4.

Glasscock ME, Schwaber MK, Nissen AJ, Jackson CG. Management of congenital ear malformations. *Ann Otol Rhinol Laryngol.* 1983;92:504.

Godoy M, Meyer R. Cirugía del pabellón auricular. Course. Presented at the *Congreso Ibero-Latinoamericano de Cirugía Plástica.* Viña del Mar, Chile, 1994.

Godoy M. Personal communication. 1990, 1994.

Goldenhar M. Associations malformatives de l'oiel et de l'oreille, en particulier le syndrome dermoide epibulbaire—appendices auriculaires—fistula auris congenita et ses relations avec la dysostose mandibulofaciale. *J Genet Hum.* 1952;1:243.

Goldwyn RM. Johann Frederick Dieffenbach (1794–1847). *Plast Reconstr Surg.* 1968;42:18.

Goleman R, Goleman B, Profeta A. Orelha em abano: aspectos evolutivos do tratamento cirárgico e tendências atuais. Presented at the *XXVII Congresso Brasilero de Chirurgia Plástica.* Rio de Janeiro, Brazil, 1990.

Gomez Montoya A, Navas E, Alvarez L. Corrección quirúrgica de las asimetrías faciales. *Cir Plast Ibero-Lat Am.* 1977;3:307.

González L. Método quirúrgico para la corrección de la hipoplasia del oído externo. In: Remorino AG, ed. *Actas del Primer Congreso Extraordinario de la Sociedad Internacional de Audiolagía.* Buenos Aires: Gillermo Kraft; 1956:1953.

Gonzalez-Ulloa M, Stevens E. Orejas en asa: prevención de alteraciones psicológicas. *Médico México.* 1960;2:77.

Gonzalez-Ulloa M. Personal communication 1989, 1990.

Gorlin RJ, Pindborg JJ, Cohen MM. *Syndromes of the Head and Neck.* New York: McGraw-Hill; 1976:546.

Gorney M. Personal communication.

Gorski M, Tarczynska IH. Surgical treatment of mandibular asymmetry. *Br J Plast Surg.* 1969;22:370.

Gradenico G. Lo sviluppo del padigliöne dell'orecchio. *Compt Rend IX Congr Int Otol Brussels.* 1888.

Granstrom G, Bergstrom K, Tjellstrom A. The bone anchored hearing aid and bone anchored epithesis for congenital ear malformations. *Otolaryngol Head Neck Surg.* 1993;109:46.

Granstrom G, Jacobsson C, Mangussom BC. Enzyme histochemical analysis of craniofacial malformations induced by retinoids. *Scand J Plast Reconstr Surg Hand Surg.* 1991;25:133.

Granstrom G, Kirkeby S. Prenatal diagnosis by isoenzymic differentiation of Treacher Collins syndrome induced by retinoids in rats. *Scand J Plast Reconstr Surg Hand Surg.* 1990;24:177.

Grenga TE. Preserving the opening after repair of split earlobes. *Plast Reconstr Surg.* 1988;82:725.

Grgicevic G. Personal communication.

Grundfast KM, Camilon F. External auditory canal stenosis and partial atresia without associated anomalies. *Ann Otol Rhinol Laryngol.* 1986;95:505.

Guilford FR, Wright WK. Secondary skin grafting of the fenestra and fenestration cavity. *Arch Otolaryngol.* 1954;64:626.

Gumener R, Bovet JL, Baudet J. Chondrite disséquante et déformante de l'oreille. *Ann Chir Plast.* 1982;27:185.

Guyuron B. Simplified harvesting of the ear cartilage graft. *Aesthetic Plast Surg.* 1986;10:37.

Hakme F, Souto AM, Kinoshita C, et al. Orelha em abano—descriçao da técnica. Presented at the *XXVII Congresso Brasileiro de Cirurgia Plástica.* Rio de Janeiro, Brazil, 1990.

Haldar A, Sharme AK, Phadke SR, Jain A, Agarwal SS. Oeis complex with craniofacial anomalies. *Defect of Blastogenesis?* 1994;15:21.

Harahap M. Repair of split earlobes. A review and new technique. *J Dermatol Surg Oncol.* 1982;8:187.

Hata Y, Hosokawa K, Yano K, Matsuka K, Ito O. Correction of congenital microtia using the tissue expander. *Plast Reconstr Surg.* 1989;84:741.

Hayashi R, Matsuo K, Hirose T. Tension lines of the auricular cartilage. *Plast Reconstr Surg.* 1991;87:869.

Hayes D. Hearing loss in infants with craneofacial anomalies. *Otolaryngol Head Neck Surg.* 1994;110:38.

Heermann H. Tympanic membrane plastic with temporal fascia. *Hals-Nasen-Ohrenh.* 1960;9:136.

Helmboltz HLF. Die mechanik der gehörknöchelchen und des trommelfells. *Pflugers Arch Ges Physiol.* 1868;1:1.

Helms J. Results of microsurgery in ear malformations. *Laryngol Rhinol Otol (Stuttg)*. 1987;66:16.

Hennekam RC, Holtus FJ, Johnson-McMillin syndrome: report of another family. *Am J Med Genet*. 1993;47:714.

Hersh JH, Ganzel TM, Fellows RA. Michel's anomaly, type I. Microtia and microdontia. *Ear Nose Throat J*. 1991;70:155.

Hinderer UT. Cirugía plástica de las deformidades de la oreja. In: *III Congreso Nacional de Cirugía Plástica*. Abstract Book (film). Valencia: 1972.

Hinderer UT. Técnica personal de otoplastía por orejas prominentes. *Noticias Médicas*. 1969;28.

Hinderer UT, del Rio JL, Fregenal FJ. Microtia. *Aesthetic Plast Surg*. 1987;11:81.

Hinderer UT, del Rio JL, Fregenal FJ. Microtia. *Plast Reconstr Surg*. 1988;82:562.

Hinderer UT, del Rio JL, Fregenal FJ. Otoplasty for lop ear. *Aesthetic Plast Surg*. 1987;11:75.

Hinderer UT, del Rio JL, Fregenal FJ. Otoplasty for lop ear. *Plast Reconstr Surg*. 1988;82:562.

Hinderer UT, del Rio JL, Fregenal FJ. Otoplasty for prominent ears. *Aesthetic Plast Surg*. 1987;11:63.

Hintzman D, Pandeya NK. Forceps in repairing torn earlobes. *Plast Reconstr Surg*. 1988;82:1106.

Hippocrates, quoted by Cowthorne T. Surgery of temporal bone. *J Laryngol Otol*. 1953;67:377.

Hirase T, Tomono T, Matsuo K. Cryptotia: our classification and treatment. *Br J Plast Surg*. 1985;38:352.

Hirase Y, Kojima T, Hirakawa H. Secondary ear reconstruction using deep temporal fascia after temporoparietal fascial reconstruction in microtia. *Ann Plast Surg*. 1990;25:53.

Hirase Y, Valauri FA, Buncke HJ. An experimental model for ear reconstruction with moulded perichondrial flaps: a preliminary report. *Br J Plast Surg*. 1989;42:223.

Hough JVD. Malformations and anatomical variations seen in the middle ear during the operation for mobilization of the stapes. *Laryngoscope*. 1958;68:1337.

House WF, Sheehy JL. Myringoplasty. *Arch Otol*. 1961;73:407.

Howard RC. The window operation for hematoma auris and perichondritis with effusion. *Laryngoscope*. 1935;45:81.

Humber PR, Kaplan IB, Horton CE. Trauma to the ear. Hematoma, laceration, amputation, and burns. In: Stark RB, ed. *Plastic Surgery of the Head and Neck*. New York: Churchill Livingstone; 1987:525.

Hurst JA, Winter RM, Baraitser M. Distinctive syndrome of short stature, craniosynostosis, skeletal changes and malformed ears. *Am J Med Genet*. 1988;29:107.

Hyakusoku H, Fumiiri M. The square flap method. *Br J Plast Surg*. 1987;40:40.

Ichinose M, Bricout N, Bach TM, Banzet P. Reparation des pertes de substance traumatiques partielles de l'oreille. *Ann Chir Plast Esthet*. 1983;28:258.

Isaac P. Otoplastías sin incisiones. Presented at the *X Congreso Ibero-Latinoamericano de Cirugía Plástica*. Viña del Mar, Chili, 1994.

Ishii H. Otoplasty. *Jpn J Plast Reconstr Surg*. 1959;3:67.

Isshiki N. Technique of total ear reconstruction with open framework, composite pseudomeatus graft, and postauricular transposition flap. In: Furnas DW, ed. *Reconstructive Surgery for Deformities of the Ear. Clin Plast Surg*. 1990;17:263.

Isshiki N, Koyama H, Suzuki S, Taira T. Surgical techniques for a deep concha, a pseudomeatus and high projection in congenital microtia. *Plast Reconstr Surg*. 1986;77:546.

Jack FL. Further observations on removal of the stapes. *Trans Am Otol Soc*. 1893;5:474.

Jackson IT. Ear reconstruction. In: Jackson, IT, ed. *Local Flaps in Head and Neck Reconstruction*. St. Louis: C.V. Mosby; 1985:262.

Jackson IT, Dubin B, Harris J. Use of contoured and stabilized conchal cartilage grafts for lower eyelid support: a preliminary report. *Plast Reconstr Surg*. 1989;83:636.

Jahn AF, Ganti F. Major auricular malformations due to accutane isotretinoin. *Laryngoscope*. 1987;97:832.

Jahrsdoerfer R. Congenital malformations of the ear, analysis of 94 operations. *Ann Otol Rhinol Laryngol*. 1980;89:348.

Jahrsdoerfer RA. Congenital atresia of the ear. *Laryngoscope*. 1978;13:1.

Jahrsdoerfer RA, Yeakley JW, Aguilar EA, Cole RR. Treacher Collins syndrome: an otologic challenge. *Ann Otol Rhinol Laryngol*. 1989;98:807.

Jahrsdoerfer R. Personal communication.

Jarvis BL, Johnson MC, Sulik KK. Congenital malformations of the external, middle, and inner ear produced by isotretinoin exposure in mouse embryos. *Otolaryngol Head Neck Surg*. 1990;102:391.

Jemec BIE. Earlobe augmentation. *Aesthetic Plast Surg*. 1986;10:35.

Jenkins AM, Finucan T. Primary nonmicrosurgical reconstruction following ear avulsion using the temporoparietal fascial island flap. *Plast Reconstr Surg*. 1989;83:148.

Joannides SV. Transcutaneous cartilage scoring for otoplasty. In: *Proceedings of the IX Congress of ISAPS*. New York: 1987:199.

Johnson PE. Otoplasty: shaping the antihelix. *Aesthetic Plast Surg.* 1994;18:71.

Jones KL, Johnson KA, Chambers CD. Offspring of women infected with varicella during pregnancy: a prospective study. *Teratology.* 1994;49:29.

Juri J, Irigari A, Juri C, Grilli D, Blanco CM, Vazquez G. Ear replantation. *Plast Reconstr Surg.* 1987;80:431.

Kaban LB, Mosés MH, Mulliken JB. Surgical correction of hemifacial microsomia in the growing child. *Plast Reconstr Surg.* 1988;82:9.

Kalimuthu R, Larson BJ, Lewis N. Earlobe repair: a new technique. *Plast Reconstr Surg.* 1984;74:299.

Kaneko T. A system for three dimensional shape measurement and its application in microtia ear reconstruction. *Keio J Med.* 1993;42:22.

Kawashima H, Ohno I, Nakaya S, Kato E, Taniguchi N. Syndrome of microtia and aortic arch anomalies resembling isotretinoin embryopathy. *J Pediatr.* 1987;111:738.

Kaye BL. A simplified auriculoplasty. In: Lewis JR Jr, ed. *The Art of Aesthetic Plastic Surgery.* Boston: Little, Brown; 1989:293.

Kessel J. Ueber das mobilisieren des steigbügels durch ausschneiden des trommelfelles, hammers und amboss bei undurchgängigkeit der tuba. *Arch Ohrenh.* 1877;13:69.

Kesselring UK, De Goumoens R. Team approach to total auricular reconstruction. *Ann Plast Surg.* 1991;26:299.

Kiesselbach W. Versuch zur anlegung eines ausseren gehorganges bei angeborener missbuldung beider ohrmusch. Mit fehlen der ausseren gehorgange. *Arch Ohrenh Lepiz.* 1882;19:127.

Kirschbaum SM. Quemaduras de la orejas. In: Kirschbaum SM, ed. *Tratamiento Integral de las Quemaduras.* Barcelona: Salvat; 1968:150.

Kisch J. Temporal muscle grafts in radical mastoid operation. *J Laryngol Otol.* 1928;43;735.

Kitchens GG. Auricular wedge resection and reconstruction. *Ear Nose Throat J.* 1989;68:673.

Kley W. Progress in tympanoplasty. *Monatsschr Ohrenh.* 1964;98:385.

Koning R, Schick U, Fucks S. Townes Brocks syndrome. *Eur J Pediatr.* 1990;150:100.

Konigsmark BW, Nager GT, Haskins HL. Recessive microtia, meatal atresia, and hearing loss. *Arch Otolaryngol.* 1972;96:105.

Koo Boo-Chai. The cleft ear lobe. *Plast Reconstr Surg.* 1961;28:681.

Kopetsky SJ. *Otologic Surgery.* New York: P.B. Hoeber; 1929:47.

Krespi YP, Pate BR Jr. Auricular reconstruction using postauricular myocutaneous flap. *Laryngoscope.* 1994;104:778.

Kristensen FW, Hesselfeldt-Nielsen J, Partoft S. Plastic surgical reconstruction in microtia, a follow-up study. *Ugeskr Laeger.* 1991;153:2568.

Kruchinsky G. Rhinoplasty with free auricle transplant. *Acta Chir Plast.* 1963;5:14.

Kruk JJ. Evaluation of surgical techniques used in treating microtia for 35 years. *Otolaryngol Pol.* 1992;46:246.

Kruk JJ. Familial occurrence of microtia. *Otolaryngology.* 1986;40:443.

Kryslova I, Fahoun J. Corrective otoplasty. *Chir Plast (Prague).* 1988;30:105.

Lambert PR. Major congenital ear malformations. Surgical management and results. *Ann Otol Rhinol Laryngol.* 1988;97:641.

Lari AA, Al-Rabah N, Dashti H. Acrobatic ears: a cause of petrified auricles. *Br J Plast Surg.* 1989;42:719.

Lassus C. Another technique for the reduction of the earlobe. *Aesthetic Plast Surg.* 1982;6:43.

Lazaro I. Personal communication.

Leber DC. Ear reconstruction. In: Georgiade NG, Georgiade GS, Riefkohl R, Barwick WJ, eds. *Essentials of Plastic, Maxillofacial, and Reconstructive Surgery.* Baltimore: Williams and Wilkins; 1987:493.

Lederer FL. Hematomas of ear. In: *Diseases of Ear, Nose and Throat,* 6th ed. Philadelphia: F.A. Davis; 1952.

Lee ST. Complications in the use of the Silastic frame for ear reconstruction. In: Maneksha RJ, ed. *Transactions of the IX International Congress of Plastic and Reconstructive Surgery.* New Delhi: McGraw-Hill; 1987:557.

Lee KJ, Hausfeld JN. Otoplasty. In: Lee KJ, ed. *Comprehensive Surgical Atlases in Otolaryngology and Head and Neck Surgery.* New York: Grune and Stratton; 1984:283.

Le Grignou P. *Agénésies de l'oreille: étude statistique sur 150 cas opérés. Analyses et commentaires.* Bordeaux: Theses; 1982:41.

Lempert J. Improvement of hearing in cases of otosclerosis: new one-stage surgical technic. *Arch Otolaryngol.* 1938;28:42.

Leng T. Fenestration of the semicircular canal for congenital microtia. *Chung-Hua-Ern-Pi-Yen-Hou-Ko-Tsa-Chih.* 1993;28:334.

Lenz W. The thalidomide syndrome. *Fortschr Med.* 1963;81:148.

Lewin ML. Correction of protruding ears by the lateral transhelical method. In: Gonzalez-Ulloa M, Meyer R, Smith JW, Zaoli G, eds. *Aesthetic Plastic Surgery.* Padova: Piccin Nuova Libraria; 1987;2:313.

Lewin ML, Argamaso RV. Cryptotia. Correction by the ear flap method. In: Gonzalez-Ulloa M, Meyer R, Smith JW, Zaoli G, eds. *Aesthetic Plastic Surgery*. Padova: Piccin Nuova Libraria; 1987;2:325.

Lewis JR. Correction of the protruding ear: principles varied depending on the type (and including a technique without incisions). Presented at the *Panel on Corrective Otoplasty*. American Society of Plastic and Reconstructive Surgeons, New York, 1967.

Lewis JS. Cancer of the ear. *Laryngoscope*. 1960;70:551.

Linstrom CJ, Meiteles LZ. Facial nerve monitoring in surgery for congenital auricular atresia. *Laryngoscope*. 1993;103:406.

Lintilhac JP. Chirugie esthetique des oreilles. In: Lintilhac JP, ed. *Du Rêve a la Réalité par la Chirugie Esthetique*. Paris: Ed. de la Table Ronde; 1945:195.

Liston SL. The relationship of the facial nerve and first branchial cleft anomalies. Embryologic considerations. *Laryngoscope*. 1982;92:1308.

Louton RB, Terranova WA. A method for external auditory canal stent fabrication. *Plast Reconstr Surg*. 1989;83:1052.

Lynberg MC, Khoury MJ, Lammer EJ, Waller KO, Cordero JF, Erickson JD. Sensitivity, specificity, and positive predictive value of multiple malformations with isotretinoin. *Teratology*. 1990;42:513.

Madzharov MM. Earlobe repair. *Plast Reconstr Surg*. 1986;77:857.

Madzharov MM. A new method of auriculoplasty for protruding ears. *Br J Plast Surg*. 1989;42:285.

Mahler D. The correction of the prominent ear. *Aesthetic Plast Surg*. 1986;10:29.

Malbec EF. Orelhas em abano: técnica operatória. A nossa experiência em 65 anos. In: Avelar JM, ed. *Cirugía plástica na infância*. Sao Paulo: Cidade Editora Cientifica; 1989:372.

Manach Y. Management of severe ear aplasias. *Acta Otorhinolaryngol Belg*. 1987;41:564.

Marini M, Lillo-Odoardi G, Fini G, Govani FA, Liberatore GM. Role of integrated imaging (computerized tomography and echography) in the surgical reconstruction of the external ear. *Radiol Med Torino*. 1993;85:394.

Marino H, Marino H Jr. A simple technique for correction of protruding ears. In: Lewis JR Jr, ed. *The Art of Aesthetic Plastic Surgery*. Boston: Little, Brown; 1989:285.

Marks MW, Argenta LC, Friedman RJ, Hall JD. Conchal cartilage and composte grafts for correction of lower lid retraction. *Plast Reconstr Surg*. 1989;83:629.

Matsuka K, Hata Y, Yano K, et al. Comparative study of auricular dimensions for the normal auricles of microtia patients, their parents, and normal individuals. *Ann Plast Surg*. 1994;32:135.

Matsumoto K. Method for reconstruction of microtia focussing on conchal creation. In: Maneksha RJ, ed. *Transactions of the IX International Congress of Plastic and Reconstructive Surgery*. New Delhi: McGraw-Hill; 1987:557.

Matsumoto K. Surgical repair of congenital earlobe cleft. *Br J Plast Surg*. 1981;34:410.

Matsumoto K, Kondoh S, Hirose T. A simple technique for reconstruction of the umbilicus, using a conchal cartilage composite graft. *Plast Reconstr Surg*. 1990;86:149.

Matsumoto K, Maeda M, Fujikawa M. Stage, laminated, costal cartilage framework for ear reconstruction. In: Furnas DW, ed. Reconstructive Surgery for Deformities of the Ear. *Clin Plast Surg*. 1990;17:273.

Matsumoto K, Maeda M, Inoue Y, Kamiji T. Reconstruction of microtia with conchal remnant. *Ann Plast Surg*. 1986;16:32.

Matsuo K, Hirose T. Reconstruction of the crus helicis in mild microtia using a preauricular tag. *Plast Reconstr Surg*. 1991;88:890.

Matsuoka A, Shitara T, Okamoto M, Furukawa K, Sano H. Cholesteatoma in children. Sex differences. *Nippon Jubiinkoka Gakkai Kaiho*. 1993;96:1430.

McCoy FJ, Macrotia. In: Masters FW, Lewis JR, eds. *Symposium on Aesthetic Surgery of the Nose, Ears, and Chin*. St. Louis: C.V. Mosby; 1973:160.

McDowell AJ. Technique, pitfalls, and complications of otoplasty. In: Masters FW, Lewis JR, eds. *Symposium on Aesthetic Surgery of the Nose, Ears, and Chin*. St. Louis: C.V. Mosby; 1973:173.

McDowell F. Successful replantation of a severed half ear. *Plast Reconstr Surg*. 1971;48:281.

Melnick M. The etiology of external ear malformations and its relation to abnormalities of the middle ear, inner ear, and other organ systems. *Birth Defects*. 1980;16:303.

Melnick M, Myrianthopoulos NC. External ear malformations: epidemiology genetics and natural history. *Birth Defects*. 1979;15:1.

Menick FJ. Artistry in aesthetic surgery—aesthetic perception and the subunit principle. *Clin Plast Surg*. 1987;14:723.

Menick FJ. Reconstruction of the ear after tumor excision. In: Furnas DW, ed. *Reconstructive Surgery for Deformities of the Ear*. Clin Plast Surg. 1990;17:405.

Mentz HA, Grahan HD, Guarisco JL. Microtia: reconstruction of the auricle. *JLA State Med Soc*. 1988;140:15.

Meurman Y, Ojala L. Primary reduction of a large operation cavity in radical mastoidectomy with muscle-periosteal flap. *Acta Oto-Laryngol.* 1949;37:245.

Meyer R. Personal communication. 1988, 1989, 1990, 1991, 1994.

Meyer R, Pellegrini P. The combined aesthetic and functional treatment of microtia. *Acta Otorhinolaryngol Ital.* 1993;13:115.

Meyer R, Sieber H. Konstruktive und rekonstruktive chirurgie des ohres. In: Gohrbandt, Gabka, Berndorfer, eds. *Handbuch der Plastische Chirurgie.* Berlin: Gruyter; 1973.

Miller CC. The surgical reduction of the excessively large ear. *Med Fort (St. Louis).* 1907;32:354.

Mills DC, Roberts W, Mason AD, McManus WF, Pruitt BA. Suppurative chondritis: its incidence, prevention and treatment. *Plast Reconstr Surg.* 1988;82:267.

Milojevic B. Aesthetic otoplasty: a new technique. *Aesthetic Plast Surg.* 1981;5:199.

Miot C. De la movilisation de l'étrier. *Rev Laryngol.* 1890;10:49,83,113,145,200.

Molina MF, Ortiz Monasterio F. Distracción mandibular en microsomia hemifacial. Presented at the *X Congreso Iberolatinoamericano de Cirugía Plástica.* Viña del Mar, Chile, 1994.

Moore JR. Correction of congenital cupping of the ear. *Chir Plastica (Berl).* 1977;4:57.

Moore MH, Hawker PB. Biointegrated hydroxylapatite coated implant fixation of facial prosthesis. *Ann Plast Surg.* 1993;31:233.

Morand SF. *Opuscules de Chirurgie.* Paris: 1768.

Morgagni, quoted by Heine B, Beck J. In: Denker A, Kahler O, eds. *Handbuch der Hals-Nasen-Ohrenheilkunde*, vol. 8. Berlín: 1927.

Moscona R, Ulman V, Har-Shai Y, Hirshowits B. Free-fat injections for the correction of hemifacial atrophy. *Plast Reconstr Surg.* 1989;84:501.

Mouly R. Scarless correction of protruding ears. *Ann Chir Plast.* 1971;16:55.

Muhlbauer W. Otopexy. In: *Proceedings of the IX Congress of ISAPS.* New York: 1987:69.

Muhlbauer WD. A simple and physiologic method to correct prominent ears. *Chir Plast.* 1972;1:126.

Muller J von. *Der Geschiteten Perlmuter-Glanzenden Fettgeschwulst, Cholesteatoma, in uber den Feimeren bau und die Formen der Krankhaften Geschwulste.* Berlin: G. Reimer; 1838:50.

Munro IR. Correction of severe facial deformity. *Can Med Assoc J.* 1975;113:531.

Munro IR, Lauritzen CGK. Classification and treatment of hemifacial microsomia. In: Caronni EP, ed. *Craniofacial Surgery.* Boston: Little, Brown; 1985:391.

Muraoka M, Nakai Y, Shimada K, Yagi H, Nakaki Y. Otoplasty in microtia. *Acta Otolaryngol Suppl (Stockh).* 1991;486:176.

Muricy JC, Marigliano RM. Otoplastia: conduta pessoal. Presented at the *XXVII Congresso Brasileiro de Cirugía Plástica*, Rio de Janeiro, Brazil, 1990.

Murray JE, Kaban LB, Mulliken JB. Analysis and treatment of hemifacial microsomia. *Plast Reconstr Surg.* 1984;74:186.

Murray JE, Kaban LB, Mulliken JB, Evans CA. Analysis and treatment of hemifacial microsomia. In: Caronni EP, ed. *Craniofacial Surgery.* Boston: Little, Brown; 1985:377.

Musgrave RH, Conklin JE. Treatment of the cauliflower ear. In: Masters FW, Lewis JR, eds. *Symposium of Aesthetic Surgery of the Nose, Ears and Chin.* St. Louis: C.V. Mosby; 1973:175.

Mustardé JC. The correction of different types of prominent ears. *Aesthetic Plast Surg.* 1983;7:163.

Mustardé JC. Effective formation of anti-helix fold without incising the cartilage. In: *Transactions of the II Congress of the International Society of Plastic Surgery.* Baltimore: Williams & Wilkins; 1960.

Mutimer KL, Banis JC, Upton J. Microsurgical reattachment of totally amputated ears. *Plast Reconstr Surg.* 1987;79:535.

Mutimer KL, Mulliken JB. Correction of cryptotia using tissue expansion. *Plast Reconstr Surg.* 1988;81:601.

Nagahama MA. Variedades de orejas prominentes. Presented at the *XX Congreso Argentino de Cirugía Plástica.* Mendoza, Argentina, 1990.

Nagata S. Modification of the stages in total reconstruction of the auricle (part I). Grafting the three dimensional costal cartilage framework for lobular type microtia. *Plast Reconstr Surg.* 1994;93:221.

Nagata S. Modification of the stages in total reconstruction of the auricle (part II). Grafting the three dimensional costal cartilage framework for concha type microtia. *Plast Reconstr Surg.* 1994;93:231.

Nagata S. Modification of the stages in total reconstruction of auricle (part III). Grafting the three dimensional costal cartilage framework for small concha-type microtia. *Plast Reconstr Surg.* 1994;93:243.

Nagata S. A new method of total reconstruction of auricle for microtia. *Plast Reconstr Surg.* 1993;92:187.

Nagata S. Secondary reconstruction for unfavorable microtia results utilizing temporoparietal and innominate fascia flaps. *Plast Reconstr Surg.* 1994;94:254.

Nakai H. Reconstruction of the helix by free composite graft from contralateral concha. *Jpn J Plast Reconstr Surg.* 1982;25:27.

Nakai H. Reconstruction of microtia with a contour accentuated framework and supplemental coverage. *Plast Reconstr Surg.* 1986;78:604.

Nakai H. Reconstruction of microtia. Pursuing a natural appearance. In: Furnas DW, ed. Reconstructive Surgery for Deformities of the Ear. *Clin Plast Surg.* 1990;17:287.

Nakai H, Ishii Y. Mechanical trauma of the ear and its reconstruction. *Jpn J Plast Reconstr Surg.* 1982;2:539.

Nakai H, Ishii Y, Nakamura S. Significance of skin coverage in total ear reconstruction. *Jpn Soc Plast Reconstr Surg Kyoto.* 1983.

Nakai H, Ishii Y, Ozaki S, Sezai Y. Use of resurfaced temporoparietalis flap in total ear reconstruction with less-than-favourable skin coverage. *Aesthetic Plast Surg.* 1984;8:253.

Nakai H, Ohmori K, Ishii Y. Problem with the lack of skin coverage in total ear reconstruction. *Jpn J Plast Reconstr Surg.* 1980;23:406.

Nakayama Y, Soeda S. Surgical treatment of Stahl's ear using the periosteal string. *Plast Reconstr Surg.* 1986;77:222.

Neumann CG. The expansion of an area of skin by progressive distention of a subcutaneous balloon: use of the method for securing skin for subtotal reconstruction of the ear. *Plast Reconstr Surg.* 1957;19:124.

Nicoletis CA. Prominent ears and flat ears. In: Lewis JR Jr, ed. *The Art of Aesthetic Plastic Surgery.* Boston: Little, Brown; 1989:299.

Nylen CO. Initiated the otomicroscope in 1921. In Shamburgh GE, ed. *Surgery of the Ear.* Philadelphia: W.B. Saunders; 1967.

Obwegeser HL. Correction of skeletal anomalies of otomandibular dysastosis. *J Maxillofac Surg.* 1974;2:73.

Ohmori S. Reconstrução auricular com uso de prótese de silicone. In: Avelar JM, ed. *Cirugía plástica na infância.* Sao Paulo: Cidade Editora Cientifica; 1989:302.

Ohmori S. Ear reconstruction. In: Maneksha RJ, ed. *Transactions of the IX International Congress of Plastic and Reconstructive Surgery.* New Delhi: McGraw-Hill; 1987:557.

Ohmori S. Macrotia and cryptotia. In: Stark RB, ed. *Plastic Surgery of the Head and Neck.* New York: Churchill Livingstone; 1987:513.

Ohmori S, Takada H. Cryptotia. *Aesthetic Plast Surg.* 1979;3:15.

Oliveira CA, Pinheiro LCF, Gomes MR. External and middle ear malformations: autosomal dominant genetic transmission. *Ann Otol Rhinol Laryngol.* 1989;98:72.

Ombredanne M. Cent opérations d'aplasie de l'oreille avec imperforation du conduit. *Acta Otorhinolaryngol.* 1957;8:315.

Oneal RM, Rohrich RJ, Izenberg PH. Skin expansion as an adjunct to reconstruction of the external ear. *Br J Plast Surg.* 1984;37:517.

Orfila D. Personal communication.

Orstavik KH, Medbo S, Mair IW. Right sided microtia and conductive hearing loss with variable expressivity in three generations. *Clin Genet.* 1990;38:117.

Orticochea M. The principle of reversal of flow in blood vessels. *Br J Plast Surg.* 1987;40:86.

Ortiz Monaterio F, Fuente AC. Early skeletal correction of hemifacial microsomia. In: Caronni EP, ed. *Craniofacial Surgery.* Boston: Little, Brown; 1985:401.

Otani H, Tanaka O, Naora H, et al. Microtia as an autosomal dominant mutation in a transgenic mouse line. A possible animal model of branchial arch anomalies. *Anat Anz.* 1991;172:1.

Pacik PT. Delayed onset of prominent ears. *Plast Reconstr Surg.* 1983;71:444.

Padgett EC. Cheek clefts (macrostomia) In: Padgett EA, ed. *Surgical Diseases of the Mouth and Jaws.* Philadelphia: W.B. Saunders; 1938:383.

Padmanabhan R. Abnormalities of the ear associated with exencephaly in mouse fetuses induced by maternal exposure to cadmium. *Teratology.* 1987;35:9.

Padmanabhan R, Hameed MS. Exencephaly and axial skeletal dysmorphogenesis induced by maternal exposure to cadmium in the mouse. *J Craniofac Genet Dev Biol.* 1986;6:245.

Page JR. Congenital bilateral microtia with total osseous atresia of the external auditory canals. Operation, and report of cases. *Trans Am Otol Soc.* 1914;13:376.

Pancoast J. *Treatise on Operative Surgery, Comprising a Description of Various Processes in the Art Including all the New Operations.* Philadelphia: Carey & Hart, G.W. Loomis; 1844.

Panse F. Pathopsychologie der entstellung. *Med Kosm.* 1958;8:229.

Parisier SC, Levenson MJ, Lucente FE. Surgical management of the external auditory canal. Course 4335. 1987 Instruction Course Program. *Otolaryngol Head Neck Surg.* 1987;96:498.

Park C. The chondrocutaneous postauricular free flap. *Plast Reconstr Surg.* 1989;84:761.

Park C, Chung S. Reverse flow post auricular arterial flap for auricular reconstruction. *Ann Plast Surg.* 1989;23:369.

Park C, Lee TJ, Shin KS, Kim YW. A single stage two-flap method of total ear reconstruction. *Plast Reconstr Surg.* 1991;88:404.

Park C, Shin KS, Kang HS, Lee YH, Lew JD. A new arterial flap from the postauricular surface: its anatomic basis and clinical application. *Plast Reconstr Surg.* 1988;82:498.

Parkash H, Grewal MS, Sidh SS. Microtia atresia with unilateral facial palsy. *Indian Pediatr.* 1982;19:445.

Parkhouse N, Evans B. Reconstruction of the ala of the nose using a composite free flap the pinna. *Br J Plast Surg.* 1985;38:306.

Parrish KL, Amedee RG. Atresia of the external auditory canal. *JLA State Med Soc.* 1990;142:9.

Pearson AA, Jacobson AD. The development of the ear. In: *Manual of the American Academy Ophthalmology and Otolaryngology.* Portland: University of Oregon Printing Department; 1967.

Peer LA. Extended use of diced cartilage grafts. *Plast Reconstr Surg.* 1954;14:178.

Peet E. The preparation of cartilage implants in ear reconstruction. In: Sanvero-Roselli G, Boggio-Rohutti G, eds. *Fourth Congress of the International Confederation for Plastic Surgery.* Rome: 1967:428.

Pelz L, Stein B. Clinical assessment of ear size in children and adolescents. *Padiatr Grenzgeb.* 1990;29:229.

Pennington DG. Discussion of "ear replantation." *Plast Reconstr Surg.* 1987;80:435.

Perroni C, Rodriguez A. Tratamiento de la oreja en asa basada en el método de Kaye. Presented at the *XVII Congreso Argentino de Cirugía Plástica—Resumenes* (abstracts), Buenos Aires, 1987.

Phelps PD, Lloyds GAS, Poswillo DE. The ear deformities in craniofacial microsomia and oculo-auriculo-vertebral displasia. *J Laryngol Otol.* 1983;97:995.

Phelps PD, Poswillo D, Lloyd GAS. The ear deformities in mandibulo-facial dysostosis (Treacher Collins syndrome). *Clin Otolaryngol.* 1981;6:15.

Pitanguy I. Personal communication, 1970, 1992.

Pitanguy I. Prominent ears. Long-term results treated by Pitanguy's technique (Portuguese). *Rev Bras Cir.* 1984;74:201.

Pitanguy I, Muller P, Kavak LK, Freitas LFP. Incisoes remodelantes no lóbulo da orelha. *Bol Cirurg Plást (Clinica Ivo Pitanguy).* 1988;78:155.

Pitanguy I, Muller P, Piccolo N, Ramalho E, Solinas R. The treatment of prominent ears: a 25 year survey of the island technique. *Aesthetic Plast Surg.* 1987;11:87.

Plester D. Myringoplasty methods. *Arch Otol.* 1963;78:310.

Politzer A. *Diseases of the Ear.* Philadelphia: Lea & Febiger; 1908.

Poncet E, Roulleau P, Peynegre R. Le problème de la plastie du pavillon dans les grandes aplasies de l'oreille. Presented at the *LXVIII Congres de la Societé Français d'O.R.L. et de Pathologie Cervico-faciale.*

Poole MD. A composite flap for early treatment of hemifacial microsomia. *Br J Plast Surg.* 1989;42:163.

Portmann M, Bebear JP, LeGrignou P. Les agénésies de l'oreille: étude analytique. *Ann Oto Laryngol.* 1983;100:403.

Poswillo D. Causal mechanisms of craniofacial deformity. *Br Med Bull.* 1975;31:101.

Poswillo DE. Discussion on Microtia: a Microform of Hemifacial Microsonia, by Bennum RD, Mulliken JB, Kaban LB, Murray JE. *Plast Reconstr Surg.* 1985;76:864.

Poswillo DE. The pathogenesis of the first and second branchial arch syndrome. *Oral Surg.* 1973;35:302.

Poswillo D. The pathogenesis of the Treacher Collins syndrome (mandibulofacial disostosis). *Br J Oral Surg.* 1975;13:1.

Powell WEM. The value of head dressings in the postoperative management of the prominent ear. *Br J Plast Surg.* 1989;42:692.

Pruzansky S. Otocranio-facial syndromes: clinical studies on mandibulofacial disostosis, hemifacial microsomia, and variants. In: Caronni EP, ed. *Craniofacial Surgery.* Boston: Little, Brown; 1985:351.

Purdue GF, Hurst JL. Chondritis of the burned ear: a preventable complication. *Am J Surg.* 1986;152:257.

Quaba A. Reconstruction of a post traumatic ear defect using tissue expansion: 30 years after Neumann. *Plast Reconstr Surg.* 1988;82:521.

Radziminski A. Remarquès sur le traitement des aplasies majeures des oreilles. *Rev Laryngol (Bord).* 1970;91:930.

Ramirez OM, Heckler FR. Reconstruction of nonmarginal defects of the ear with chondrocutaneous advancement flaps. *Plast Reconstr Surg.* 1989;84:32.

Raulo Y. Treacher Collins syndrome: analysis and principles of surgery. In: Caronni EP, ed. *Craniofacial Surgery.* Boston: Little, Brown; 1985:371.

Richards CS. Middle ear changes in rubella deafness. *J Otol Soc Aust.* 1963;1:173.

Richier, cited by Senechal and Pech. *Chirugie du Pavillon de l'Oreille.* Paris: Arnette; 1970:96.

Rijavek MC. Personal communication.

Rogers BO. Book review. Aesthetic and reconstructive otoplasty, by Davis, J. *Aesthetic Plast Surg.* 1987;11:128.

Rogers BO. Commentary. In: McDowell F, ed. *The Sourcebook of Plastic Surgery.* Baltimore: Williams & Wilkins; 1977:348, 353.

Rogers BO. Commentary. In: McDowell F, ed. *The Sourcebook of Plastic Surgery.* Baltimore: Williams & Wilkins; 1977:353.

Rogers BO. Developmental defects of the ear. Normal and abnormal positioning of the external ear. In: Stark RB, ed. *Plastic Surgery of the Head and Neck.* New York: Churchill Livingstone; 1987:467.

Rogers BO. Embryology and fetal development of the ear. In: Stark RB, ed. *Plastic Surgery of the Head and Neck.* New York: Churchill Livingstone; 1987:463.

Rogers BO. Hippolyte Morestin (1869–1919), part I, a brief biography. *Aesthetic Plast Surg.* 1982;6:141.

Rogers BO. Julius von Szymanowski (1829–1868). His life and contributions to plastic surgery. *Plast Reconstr Surg.* 1979;64:465.

Rogers BO. A medical "first": Ely's operation to correct protruding ears. *Aesthetic Plast Surg.* 1987;11:71.

Rogers BO. A medical "first": Ely's operation to correct protruding ears. *Plast Reconstr Surg.* 1988;82:562.

Rogers BO. Reconstruction of the auricle (Rekonstrukce Boltce) by Ladislav Barinka. Book review. *Aesthetic Plast Surg.* 1990;14:79.

Rogers BO. Personal communication.

Rojas GG. Auriculoplastías mediante plicatura transfixionante percutanea del antihelix. Presented at the *XX Congreso Argentino de Cirugía Plástica.* Mendoza, Argentina, 1990.

Rojas GG. Personal communication, 1990, 1994.

Rollnick BR, Kaye CI, Nagatoshi K, Hauck W, Martin AO. Oculoauriculovertebral dysplasia and variants. Phenotypic characteristics of 294 patients. *Am J Med Genet.* 1987;26:361.

Rosa FW, Wilk AL, Kelsey FO. Teratogen update: vitamin A congeners. *Teratology.* 1986;33:355.

Ross DF, Vallino LD, Galloway D, Keller P. Modification of the traditional bone conduction hearing aid. *Cleft Palate Craneofac. J.* 1993;30:328.

Ross JK, Matti B, Davies DM. A Silastic foam dressing for the protection of the postoperative ear. *Br J Plast Surg.* 1987;40:213.

Ross RB. Lateral facial dysplasia (first and second branchial arch syndrome, hemifacial microsomia). *Birth Defects.* 1975;11:51.

Rothfeld ID. Methods of otoplasty. Course 4113. *Otolaryngol Head Neck Surg.* 1987;96:487.

Ruder RO. New concept in microtia repair. *Arch Otolaryngol Head Neck Surg.* 1988;114:1016.

Rueckert F, Brown FE, and Tanzer RC. Overview of experience of Tanzer's group with microtia. *Clin Plast Surg.* 1990;17:223.

Rueckert F, Brown FE. Developmental defects of the ear. Microtia. In: Stark RB, ed. *Plastic Surgery of the Head and Neck.* New York: Churchill Livingstone; 1987:488.

Rüedi L. The surgical treatment of atreis auris congenita: a clinical and histological report. *Trans Am Laryngol Rhinol Otol Soc.* 1954;373.

Saito R, Matsumura M, Takata N, Ogura Y, Iwahori N, Hoshimo K. Histopathologic study of congenital auris atresia in the human embryo. *Arch Otolaryngol.* 1981;107:215.

Salvatori C. Personal communication.

Sarrat R. Desarrollo evolutivo y embriológico de la región facial. *Cir Plast Ibero-Lat Am.* 1975;1:203.

Sasaki GH. Discussion. Correction of congenital microtia using the tissue expander (Hata, Hosokawa, Yano, Matsuka and Ito). *Plast Reconstr Surg.* 1989;84:752.

Sasaki GH. Tissue expansion. An alternative method for the reconstruction of major acquired and congenital ear deformities, ear reconstruction. Guidelines and case analyses. Dow Corning Wright booklet, 1988.

Sasaki GH. Tissue expansion in reconstruction of acquired auricular defects. In: Furnas DW, ed. Reconstructive Surgery for Deformities of the Ear. *Clin Plast Surg.* 1990;17:327.

Satch R. Morphology of the auricles: observation of postnatal changes in shape of auricles. *Jpn J Plast Reconstr Surg.* 1986;29:610.

Sawada Y, Nakajima T, Yoshimura Y. Auricular composite graft from the scapha and its repair using a retroauricular subcutaneous pedicle flap. *Aesthetic Plast Surg.* 1987;11:53.

Sbitany U, Caldwell EH. Treatment of a giant congenital hairy nevus of the ear. *Plast Reconstr Surg.* 1986;78:242.

Scheibe A. Doppelseitige kongenitale atresie des gehörgangs. *München Med Wchnschr.* 1904;51:88.

Schewe EJ, Pappalardo C. Cancer of the external ear. *Am J Surg.* 1962;104:753.

Schuffenecker J, Reichert H. Notre expérience â propos de 3200 corrections d'oreilles proéminentes par modifications deslignes de force selon le procédé de Reichert. *Ann Chir Plast.* 1982;27:334.

Schuknecht HF. Congenital aural atresia. *Laryngoscope.* 1989;99:908.

Schulhof E, Valdez G. Pathology and therapeutics of the perforated ear drum. *Franco Am Med Assoc.* 1944; Aug. 3.

Schultz RC. Surgically produced cleft palates in rabbits. A study of resulting middle ear infections. *Plast Reconstr Surg.* 1964;33:120.

Schwaber M, Glasscock M, Nissen A, Jackson CG. The place of fenestration in congenital ear surgery. *Am J Otol.* 1983;4:222.

Schwartze H. Ueber erworbene atresie und strictur des gehörganges und deren behandlung. *Arch Ohrenh.* 1899;47:71.

Senechal G, Lamas G, Soudant J, Senechal B. Traitment des sténoses acquises du conduit auditif externe. Intérêt des lambeaux pédiculés. *Ann Chir Plast Esthet.* 1988;33:342.

Shambaugh GE Jr. Primary skin graft in modified (Bondy) radical mastoidectomy for preservation of hearing in cases of genuine cholesteatoma. *Arch Otolaryngol.* 1936;23:222.

Shambaugh GE Jr. The surgical treatment of meningitis of otitic and nasal origin. *JAMA.* 1937;108:696.

Shambaugh GE Jr, Derlacki EL. Primary skin grafting of the fenestra and fenestration cavity. *Arch Otolaryngol.* 1956;64:46.

Shea JJ. Vein graft closure of eardrum perforations. *J Laryngol Otol.* 1960;74:358.

Sheehy JL. Tympanic membrane grafting. *Laryngoscope.* 1964;74:985.

Sherman JE, Bromley GS. Shell ear and satyr ear. In: Stark RB, ed. *Plastic Surgery of the Head and Neck.* New York: Churchill Livingstone; 1987:518.

Siegert R, Weerda H, Hoffmann S, Mohadjer C. Clinical and experimental evaluation of intermittent intraoperative short term expansion. *Plast Reconstr Surg.* 1993;92:248.

Simons G, Legray P, Darsonval V, Greco JM. La réparation du lobe auriculaire fendu. *Ann Chir Plast.* 1980;5:139.

Skoog T. Protruding ears. In: Skoog T, ed. *Plastic Surgery.* Stockholm: Almquist and Wiksell International; 1974:251.

Smahel Z. Craniofacial changes in hemifacial microsomia. *J Craniofac Genet Dev Biol.* 1986;6:151.

Smahel J, Converse JM. Anatomical features of auricular and retroauricular skin. *Chir Plast.* 1980;5:139.

Smahel Z, Theuer J. Interrelations between the involvement of individual branchiogenic components in microtia. *J Craniofac Genet Dev Biol.* 1986;6:139.

Song R. Reconstrucão auricular num único tempo cirúrgico? In: Avelar JM, ed. "Cirugía plástica na infância." Sao Paulo: Cidade Editora Cientifica; 1989:327.

Song YG, Zhuang HX. One stage total reconstruction of the ear simultaneous tympanoplasty. *Clin Plast Surg.* 1990;17:251.

Sorin E, Davis JE. Timpanotomía superior en las malformaciones auriculares congénitas. Presented at the *Bol. Society of Argentina ORL,* Buenos Aires: June 9, 1976.

Souza A.M. Correção de orelhas em abano por duas vias de acesso. In: Avelar JM, ed. *Cirugía Plástica na infância,* Sao Paulo: Cidade Editora Cientifica; 1989:379.

Stagnaro EJ, Manassero R. Colgajo de fascia temporoparietal para la reconstrucción auricular. Presented at the *XVII Congreso Argentino de Cirugía Plástica.* Resúmenes (abstracts), Buenos Aires, 1987.

Stark RB. *Plastic Surgery of the Head and Neck.* New York: Churchill Livingstone; 1987.

Stark RB. Otoplasty for prominent ears. General methods. In: Stark, RB, ed. *Plastic Surgery of the Head and Neck.* New York: Churchill Livingstone; 1987.

Stark RB. Cleft ear lobule. In Stark RB, ed. *Plastic Surgery of the Head and Neck.* New York: Churchill Livingstone; 1987:532.

Stark RB, Saunders DE. Otoplasty. In: Stark RB, ed. *Aesthetic Plastic Surgery.* Boston: Little, Brown; 1980:345.

Stewart JM, Downs MP. Congenital conductive hearing loss. The need for early identification and intervention. *Pediatrics.* 1993;91:355.

Storck R. Orelhas em abano. In: Avelar JM, ed. *Cirugía plástica na infância,* Sao Paulo: Ciudade Editora Cientifica; 1989:384.

Strauch B, Sharzer LA, Petro J, Greenstein B. Replantation of amputated parts of the penis, nose, ear and scalp. *Clin Plast Surg.* 1983;10:115.

Strisciuglio P, Ballabio A, Parenti G. Microtia with meatal atresia and conductive deafness: mild and severe manifestations within the same sibship. *J Med Genet.* 1986;23:459.

Sugino H, Tsuzuki K, Bandoh Y, Tange I. Surgical correction of Stahl's ear using the cartilage turnover and rotation method. *Plast Reconstr Surg.* 1989;83:160.

Suzuki J, Suzuki M, Kodera K, Kaga K. Transplants and implants for anomalies. *Acta Otorhinolaryngol (Belg).* 1988;42:784.

Sylven B, Hamberger CA. Malignant melanoma of the external ear. *Ann Otol Rhinol Laryngol.* 1950;59:631.

Tabb HG. Closure of perforations of the tympanic membrane by vein grafts. *Laryngoscope.* 1960;73:699.

Takato T. First branchial cleft sinus in the first and second arch syndrome. *Jpn J Plast Reconstr Surg.* 1988;8:359.

Tan KH. Long-term survey of prominent ear surgery: a comparison of two methods. *Br J Plast Surg.* 1986;39:270.

Tanaka Y, Tajima S. Completely successful replantation of an amputated ear by microvascular anastomosis. *Plast Reconstr Surg.* 1989;84:665.

Tanino R, Miyasaka M. Reconstruction of microtia using tissue expander. *Clin Plast Surg.* 1990;17:339.

Tanzer RC. The correction of microtia. In: Brent B, Brent BP, eds. *The Artistry of Reconstructive Surgery.* St. Louis: C.V. Mosby; 1987:93.

Tanzer RC. Discussion of Silastic framework complications. In: Tanzer RC, Edgerton MT, eds. *Symposium on Reconstruction of the Auricle*. St. Louis: C.V. Mosby; 1974:87.

Tanzer RC. The reconstruction of acquired defects of the ear. *Plast Reconstr Surg.* 1965;35:355.

Tanzer RC. Total reconstruction of the external ear. *Ann Plast Surg.* 1983;10:76.

Tanzer RC. Personal communication, 1988.

Teizen IC, Almeida MAF, Almeida SS. Cartilagen autógena ou prótese de silicone na reconstruçào total de orelha. Presented at the *XXVII Congresso Brasileiro de Cirurgía Plástica*. Rio de Janeiro: Brazil; 1990.

Thomson HG, Correa A. Unilateral microtia reconstruction. Is the position symmetrical? *Plast Reconstr Surg.* 1993;92:852.

Thomson HG, Winslow J. Microtia reconstruction: does the cartilage framework grow? *Plast Reconstr Surg.* 1989;84:908.

Tjellström A. Osseointegrated implants for replacement of absent or defective ears. In: Furnas DW, ed. Reconstructive Surgery for Deformities of the Ear. *Clin Plast Surg.* 1990;17:355.

Tolleth H. A hierarchy of values in design and construction of ear. In: Furnas DW, ed. Reconstructive Surgery for Deformities of the Ear. Clin Plast Surg. 1990;17:193.

Toynbee J. *Diseases of the Ear*. London: 1860.

Toynbee J. Pathological and surgical observations on the diseases of the ear. *Medico Chir Trans.* 1841;24:190.

Trias AA, Semenaro C, Pesqueira T. Otoplasty: personal variations on Skoog's technique. Presented at the *XI Biennial Congress, International Society of Aesthetic Plastic Surgery*, Jalisco: Mexico; 1992.

Turpin IM. Microsurgical replantation of the external ear. In: Furnas DW, ed. Reconstructive Surgery for Deformities of the External Ear. *Clin Plast Surg.* 1990;17:397.

Upton J, Mulliken JB, Hicks PD, Murray JE. Restoration of the facial contour using free vasculared omentum transfer. *Plast Reconstr Surg.* 1980;66:560.

Valvassori GE. Discussion, remarks. Preoperative tomography in congenital malformations of the ear. *Trans Am Acad Ophthalmol Otolaryngol.* 1966;70:59.

Vecchione TR. Needle scoring of the anterior surface of the cartilage in otoplasty. *Plast Reconstr Surg.* 1979;64:568.

Veintemillas F. Métodos autoplásticos para la restauración quirúrgica de la agenesia auditiva. *Rev Brasil Oto-Rino-Laring Sao Paulo.* 1940.

Ver Meulen VR. Macrotia the oversized ear: method of reduction. *Laryngoscope.* 1970;80:1053.

Verloes A. Hypertelorism-microtia-clefting syndrome. *Genet Couns.* 1994;5:283.

Wallace AF. History of plastic surgery. *J R Soc Med.* 1978;7:834.

Warszawer-Schvarcz L. The use of color-head straight pins for prominent ear correction. *Aesthetic Plast Surg.* 1980;4:303.

Wellisz T. The ear model: an aid for total ear reconstruction. *Plast Reconstr Surg.* 1988;82:1079.

Wellisz TZ, Cutting CB, McCarthy JG. The effects of unilamellar perichondrial dissection on the growth of rabbit ear. *Plast Reconstr Surg.* 1987;79:935.

Welsh F. Otoplasty: excision of conchal floor cartilage. *Aesthetic Plast Surg.* 1980;4:87.

Wilkes GH, Wolfaardat JF. Osseointegrated alloplastic versus, autogenous ear reconstruction: criteria for treatment selection. *Plast Reconstr Surg.* 1994;93:967.

Wilmot TJ. Hereditary conductive deafness due to incusstapes abnormalities and associated wtih pinna deformity. *J Laryngol Otol.* 1970;84:469.

Wolach B, Raas-Rothschild A, Metzker A, et al. Skin mastocytosis with short stature, conductive hearing loss and microtia. A new syndrome. *Clin Genet.* 1990;37:64.

Wolfe MM. Protruding ears: the psychological effect and plastic correction. *Med Rec NY.* 1936;114:306.

Wolfsberg EA, Grigbsy TM. Rokitansky sequence in association with facio-auricular-vertebral sequences: part of a mesodermal malformation spectrum? *Am J Med Genet.* 1990;17:100.

Wright WK. Tissues for tympanic grafting. *Arch Otol.* 1963;78:291.

Wright WR. Otoplasty goals and principles. *Arch Otolaryngol.* 1970;92:568.

Wullstein H. Funktionelle Operationen im Mittelohr mit Hilfe des frein Spalt-Fappen-Trans. *Plantatis Arch Ohren-Nassen-u Kehlkopfh.* 1952;161:422.

Wynn SK. On the article "Reconstruction of a Traumatic Subtotal Ear Loss with Two Skin Tubes." *Plast Reconstr Surg.* 1971;49:332.

Yamaguchi N, Sando I, Hashida Y, Takahashi H, Matsune S. Histologic study of eustachian tube cartilage with and without congenital anomalies. A preliminary study. *Ann Otol Rhinol Laryngol.* 1990;99:984.

Yanai A, Fukuda O, Nagata S, Tanaka H. A new method utilizing the bipedicle flap for reconstruction of the external auditory canal in microtia. *Plast Reconstr Surg.* 1985;76:464.

Yanai A, Fukuda O, Yamada A. Problems encountered in contouring a reconstructed ear of autogenous cartilage. *Plast Reconstr Surg.* 1985;75:185.

Yanai A, Tange I, Bandoh Y, Tsuzuki K, Sugino H, Nagata S. Our method of correcting cryptotia. *Plast Reconstr Surg.* 1988;82:965.

Yoel J. Parotid aplasia. In: Yoel J, ed. *Pathology and Surgery of the Salivary Glands.* Springfield: Charles C. Thomas; 1975:136.

Yoshimura Y, Nakajima T, Kami T. Scalp graft for elevation of the reconstructed auricle. *Plast Reconstr Surg.* 1987;80:352.

Zankl M, Zang KD. Inheritance of microtia and aural atresia in a family with 5 affected members. *Clin Genet.* 1979;16:331.

Zaoli G, Otoplasty. In Gonzalez-Ulloa M, Meyer R, Smith J, Zaoli G, eds. *Aesthetic Plastic Surgery.* Padova: Piccin Nuova Libraria; 1987;2:165.

Zenteno S. Expansor en reconstruccion auricular. Presented at the *XXVII Congresso Brasileiro de Cirurgía Plástica*, Rio de Janeiro, Brazil, 1990.

Zenteno S. Expansores en auriculoplastias. Presented at the *XX Congreso Argentino de Cirugía Plástica*, Mendoza, Argentina, 1990.

Zhou G. One stage reconstruction of microtia associated with hemifacial soft tissue aplasia. *Chung Hua Cheng Hsing Shao Shang Wai Ko Tsa Chin.* 1990;6:20.

Zlotogora J, Eidelman A, Dudin A, Voss R. Microtia in infants with chromosomal trisomy. *J Craniofac Genet Dev Biol.* 1988;8:205.

Zöllner F. The principles of plastic surgery of the sound-conducting apparatus. *J Laryngol Otol.* 1955;69:637.

Zoltán J. Reconstruction of auricular skin. Reconstructive procedures of the auricle and in its neighborhood. In: Zoltán J, ed. *Atlas of Skin Repair.* München: Kaeger-Basel; 1984:160.

Zoltie N. Split earlobes. A method of repair preserving the hole. *Plast Reconstr Surg.* 1987;80:619.

Zong-Ji C, Xian-Lun W. One stage total auricle reconstruction. *Clin Med J.* 1985;98:13.

Zuang HX. Treatment of congenital microtia. *Chung Hua Cheng Hsing Shao Shang Wai Ko Tsa Chin.*, 1988;4:17.

Index

—a—

Aesthetic otoplasty, 3–23
 and conchal flap, 9
 cryptotia and satyr ear, 10–13
 and healing potential, 19
 and keloids, 19–22
 secondary otoplasty, 3–9
 and test for measurement of delicacy, 23
 and trauma, 13–19
Aesthetic surgery, 66
Age, and covering neotympanic membrane, 96
Allogen material, 101
Alveolo-ectodermal membrane, branchia as, 25
Anatomy
 defined, 66
 muscle layer and, 70
Anotic cartilage, 115
Anterior approach, 88
Anterior auricle, 83
Anthelical cauda, 85
Antia, N. H., 9
Antitragus, 5, 7, 8
Appositional growth of cartilage, 46
Artery, stapedial, 28
Articular surfaces, cartilage in, 44
Atresia
 auricular, 34–35, 66
 bilateral, 101–110
 operating on unilateral, 33–34
 otologic criteria for reconstruction, 33
 partial, 35, 36–42
 and PPC syndrome, 59
 total, 63–65, 86–87, 111–114
 unilateral, 32–33
Atresic plate, 87–88, 91, 92, 94

Audiometric tests, after meatomyringoplasty, 98–99
Audiometry, after surgery for moderate microtia and total atresia, 65
Auditory acuity, 102
Auricle
 anterior, 83
 development of, 30
 partial atresia syndromes and, 37
 subtotal avulsion of, 14
Auricular atresia, 34–35, 66
 total, 86–87
Auricular cartilage, 43, 45–46, 102, 106
Auricular cartilage framework, 115
Auricular chondo-graft, growth of, 81–82
Auricular dysmorphia, 24
Auricular functional properties, 54–58
 bioimmunologic reactions, 57
 in Chinese medicine, 57–58
 organ of delicacy, 57
 organ of mobility, 56
 organ of sensation, 55–56
 reflex defense, 56
 skeletal formation of, 55
 skin color, 57
 skin function, 56–57
 sound reception, 55
 in surgery, 58
 trophic (growth, healing), 56
Auricular "halo," 9
Auricular integument, 68–71
 covering and, 68–69
 lobule and, 69–70
 muscle layer and, 70–71
 reinnervation and, 71

Auricularis muscles
 posterior, 6
 superioris, 10, 11
Auricular movement, Davis test and, 71
Auricular skeletal support, reconstruction and, 54
Auricular SMAS, 86
Auricular structures, 24
Auricular tissue texture delicacy, 23
Auriculoplasty, 114. *See also* Otoplasty
 lobule and, 69–70
 for moderate microtia and total atresia, 63–65
 nerve supply recovery in, 19
 radical, 66–100
Autograft, 54

—b—

Bald skin. *See* Skin grafts
Beta therapy, 22
Bilateral atresia, 101–110
 framework, 104–106
 otologic considerations, 103
 upper nubbin, 104
Bilateral microtia, 101–110
 corrected with auricular cartilage, 106
 repaired with microtial cartilage on same side, 107–110
Bioimmunologic reactions, 57
Bleeding, in otoplasty, 6
Bone, tympanic, 41–42
Bone graft
 in helical sulcus surgery, 73–74
 in meatomyringoplasty, 89
Branchia, development of, 25–26
Branchial apparatus concepts,

analysis of, 25–31
Branchial arches, 26
   embryo organic derivatives from first, 26–27
   embryo organic derivatives from second, 27
Branchial circulation, 28
Brent, Burton, 105
"Bud that blooms" expansion chondroplasty, 108

—c—

Canal, construction after auriculoplasty, 102–103
Canal, 35–36, 92. *See also* Unilateral atresia; Unilateral microtia
   auricular atresia and, 34–35
   flaps and grafts in, 39–41
   and helical sulcus, 75
   late strictures of reconstructed, 99
   partial atresia syndromes and, 37
   secondary strictures of reconstructed, 99
   in stereotactic surgery, 89
Canal cartilage atresia, 87
Candás, Oscar, 31, 32, 89
Canoe ear, 63, 108
Cartilage, 6, 43–52, 68, 115. *See also* Microtial cartilage
   auricular, 69
   auricular (elastic), 43
   and auricular functional properties, 54–58
   basic considerations in, 44
   in bilateral atresia, 103
   conchal, 6, 7
   elastic, 45–46
   fibrous, 45
   for framework in bilateral atresia, 104–106
   for framework material, 101–102
   grafting of rabbit, 47–54
   graft of, 7
   Grgicevic's investigation of, 46–47
   histogenesis, growth, and regeneration of, 46
   hyaline (costal), 43, 45
   nutrition of, 44–45
   scaphal, 6
   white fibrocartilage, 44
   yellow elastic, 44

Cartilaginous hillocks, 24
Cartilaginous viscerocranium, 29
Cervical flap, and helical sulcus, 75
Chinese medicine, 57
Cholesteatoma, 34
Chondo-SMAS repair, 72
Chondrocutaneous flap, 67
Chondro-graft growth, 81–82
Chondroplasty, expansion, 102, 108
Chondrotomy, expansion, 105, 115
Cigarette smoking. *See* Smoking
Clinical dysmorphia, 24
Collagen, in cartilage, 44
Complexes, ear inferiority complex as, 2
Computed tomography (CT) scans, 32
Conchal cartilage, 113
   reconstruction and, 15
   trauma and, 13
Conchal cartilage floor, 6, 7
Conchal cavity, reduction of, 7–8
Conchal flap, 9–13
Conchal skin, 22
Conchal wall, 5, 6
Condylar neck fracture, 14
Congenital canal atresia, 36
Congenital cholesteatoma, 34
Congenital microtia and atresia, stereotactic surgery for, 97
Converse, John, 17
Costal (hyaline) cartilage. *See* Hyaline (costal) cartilage
Covering. *See also* Skin covering; Skin grafts
   and auricular integument, 68–69
   of neotympanic membrane, 94–98
Cranial development, 28–29
Crossed bite, 14
Crus, 4, 5, 6, 8
Cryptotia
   mechanism of, 11
   and satyr ear, 10–13
CT scans. *See* Computed tomography (CT) scans
Cutaneous layer, 30

—d—

Davis, J., 24, 29, 30, 45
Davis syndrome, 37
Davis tests, 10

auricular movement and, 71
microtia and, 72
SMAS contracture test and, 105
Defective tympanic bone-SMAS, 30
Defects, categorizing, 3–5
Deformity
   early recognition of, 32
   moderate microtia and total atresia, 63–65
   pinna-partial canal (PPC) syndrome and, 58
   secondary rhinoplasty surgical procedure for, 3–9
Delicacy
   of auricle, 57
   measurement of, 23
Diagnosis
   of atresia, 34
   by plastic surgeon, 66
Diamante, Vicente, 31–32, 88, 89
Dieffenbach, Johann, 17
Discriminitive (double pinpoint expansion) test, 78
Dissection, in otoplasty, 6
Dog, ear reconstruction on, 2
Donor ear, 67
Dressing, after otoplasty, 7
Dysgenesis, 24

—e—

Ear. *See also* External ear; Middle ear
   embryology of external, 24
   loss and replacement of, 15–19
Ear cartilage, 115
Ear inferiority complex, 2
Ear-to-head relationship, 8
Education of the Virgin (painting), 23
Elastic cartilage. *See* Auricular cartilage
Electronic microscopy, 115
Embryology, of external ear, 24, 67
Embryo organic derivatives
   cranial development, 28–29
   from first branchial arch, 26–27
   from second branchial arch, 27
   stapedial artery, 28
   tympanic ring, 29–31
Endodermic mucosa layer, 30
Epicritic (cotton wool test), 78
Epicritic (cotton wool test) sensation, 61

Epithelium. *See also* Skin grafts
   in auricular area, 68
Expansile framework, 105
Expansion chondroplasty, 102, 108
Expansion chondrotomy, 105, 115
External auditory canal, 30
External aural canal, construction
   in congenital ear atresia, 89–94
External auricular canal, 30, 31
External ear
   embryology of, 24, 67
   physiology of, 67
   relationship with middle ear, 35

–f–

Facial nerve, and helical sulcus
   surgery, 75
Fascia tissue formation, 11
Fenestration technique, 92
Fetus, cranial development in, 28
Fibrous cartilage, 45
Fibrous mesodermic layer, 30
Fibrous pseudocapsule, 43
First and second arch syndrome, 66
First branchial arch, 26–27
Fisch, Ugo, 32
Fistula
   single-tract, 36–37
   and skin grafts, 96
Flaps. *See* Skin flaps
Fossa triangularis, 4
Framework, and bilateral atresia,
   104–106
Framework material, 101–102
Frontalis muscle, 10
Functional anatomy, 30
Functional auriculoplasty, 114

–g–

Gillies, 114
Gradenico, G., 24
Grafting, 7, 15, 17–18. *See also*
   Cartilage; Skin grafts
   of cartilage, 46–55
   with homo-grafts, necro-grafts,
      and allogen material, 101
   of hyaline (costal) cartilage, 43
   for PPC syndrome, 59, 60
Grgicevic, Gustavo, 24, 32, 36, 37,
   46–47
Growth, 56
   of cartilage, 46

–h–

Hair, 111
Hairless skin. *See* Skin grafts
Healing, 19–22, 56
   and covering neotympanic membrane, 96–97
   after helical sulcus surgery, 74, 75
   and keloids, 19–22
Hearing loss, 102
   and bilateral atresia, 103
Helical dome
   curve, 10
   revision, 17, 19
Helical drape, 10
Helical skin, keloid and, 22
Helical sulcus, 72–86
   and absent tragus, 84
   and bilateral atresia, 104–105
   chondro-graft growth and, 81–82
   late deepening of, 84–85
   late revision for, 82–84
   second operation on, 74
   surgical sequence for, 73–80
Helix, 6, 9
Helix-mastoid prominence, 8
Hemifacial microsomia, 66,
   111–114
   correction of, 75
High-resolution computed tomography (HRCT), 32, 91, 115
High-resolution light microscopy,
   115
Hillocks, 24
His, Wilhelm, 24
Histogenesis, of cartilage, 46
Homo-grafts, 101
HRCT. *See* High-resolution computed tomography (HRCT)
Hyaline (costal) cartilage, 43, 44,
   45. *See also* Grafting; Skin grafts
   for framework material, 101–102
   grafting of, 54
Hyperbaric oxygenation, 17

–i–

Infection, in atresic patient, 34
Inferiority complexes, 2
Inguinal skin graft, 105. *See also*
   Skin grafts
Instruments, for obtaining skin covering, 68–69
Integument, auricular, 68–71

Internal maxillary arches, 27
Interstitial growth, of cartilage, 46
Intrauterine microsurgery, 115

–j–

Jahrsdoerfer, Robert, 32
Juxtatympanic pouch, 35, 37, 91
   in total auricular artresia, 86

–k–

Keloids, 19–22
Kirkham method, 84

–l–

Lagos, Nestor Ruben, 47
La Tour, George de, 23
Llorca, O., 28
Lobule, 9
   and auricular integument, 69–70
Lower ear, formation of, 15–16

–m–

Magnetic resonance, 115
Malleus manubrium, 92
Mandibular asymmetry, 66, 113
Mastoid. *See* Stereotactic surgery
Mastoid fascia, 6
Maxillofacial surgery, 14
Measurement, by plastic surgeon,
   67
Meatomyringoplasty, 88–89, 98–99,
   113. *See also* Neotympanic
   membrane; Stereotactic surgery
   for moderate microtia and total
      atresia, 63–65
Mesoderm, 29
Methods, selecting, 115
Microphotography, 115
Microscopy, 115
Microsomia, 113
   hemifacial, 66, 111–114
Microsurgery, 115
Microtia, 3. *See also* Bilateral microtia
   and auricular atresia, 31–33
   Davis tests and, 72
   moderate, 24–42, 63–65
   peanut, 111–114
   severe, 66–100
   unilateral, 32–33, 37–42, 67–68
Microtia-atresia-microsomia, as one
   syndrome, 115

Microtia-atresia repair, 32
Microtial cartilage, 102, 106
   and bilateral atresia, 105
   repairing severe microtia with, 107–110
Middle ear
   atresic, 33–34
   relationship with external ear, 35
Middle ear chronic disease, 34
Middle ear elevators, 6
Mobility, auricle and, 56
Moderate microtia, 24–42, 63–65
Mucosa, 92, 93, 94
Mulcahy, Jorge, 1
Muscle layer, and auricular integument, 70–71
Muscular contraction, 10
Myringoplasty, in auricular atresia, 66

—n—

Necro-grafts, 101
Needles with dye, in otoplasty, 6
Neolobe sandwich method, 77–78
Neotympanic membrane, covering, 94–98
Nerve, facial, 75
Nerve supply, recovery in auriculoplasty, 19
Neurocranium, 29
Neuroendocrine medication, 22
Noden, 26
Nubbin. See Upper nubbin
Nutrition, for cartilage, 44–45

—o—

Orfila, Daniel, 31
Ossification, 89
   tympanic, 87
Osteotomy, 38–42
Otitis media, 33–34
Otoplasty. See also Aesthetic otoplasty
   aesthetic, 3–23
Otosurgery, 115

—p—

Parotid deficiency, 66
Parotid depression, 113
Partial atresia, 24–42
   syndromes, 36–42
   and total atresia, 35

Patient, importance of, 1–2
Peanut microtia, 78
   correction of, 111–114
Peet, E., 114
Perichondrium, 6
Pharyngeal membranes, 26
Pharyngeal pouches, 26, 27
Pharyngeal sulci, 26
Physiologic embryology, 30
Physiology, of external ear, 67
Pinna dysmorphism, 36
Pinna-partial canal (PPC) syndrome, 30, 58–62
   case study of, 59–62
   characteristics of, 62
   skin flap in, 59
Plastic surgery, 115
   justification of, 66–67
Plastic surgery anatomy, 66
Plug resorption, 87
Pneumatization, 87–88
Postauricular sulcus, surgical procedure and, 74
Posterior approach, 88
Postoperative condition
   after cryptotia and satyr ear surgery, 13
   after ear reconstruction surgery, 17
   after PPC syndrome surgery, 60
   smoking and, 17
Postoperative course, after otoplasty, 7
Posttraumatic keloid pathology, 20–22
PPC syndrome. See Pinna-partial canal (PPC) syndrome
Pre-endaural approach, 115
Preoperative condition, for cryptotia and satyr ear, 13
Prepuce skin graft, 95
Pseudocapsule, 43
Ptotic antitragus, 5

—r—

Rabbit cartilage, in grafting, 47–54
Radix, repositioning, 9
Reconstruction
   autograft and, 54
   for ear loss, 15–19
Reflex defense, auricle and, 56
Regeneration, of cartilage, 46

Reichert's cartilage, 27
Reinnervation, auricular integument and, 71
Reossification, 99
Retroaural sulcus, grafting to, 111
Rhinoplasty. See also Otoplasty
   secondary, 3
Rhytidectomy, 16
Rib cartilage, 101, 108
Rodriguez, A. Ferrer, 24
Rogers, Blair, 17
Roof atresia, 30
Rosler, José, 89

—s—

Salvatori, Carlos, 32
Satyr ear, 4
   cryptotia and, 10–13
Scapha, 9
   insufficient, 4
Scaphal cartilage, 6
Scaphoid fossa deficiency, 10
Scarring, 17. See also Skin grafts
   and helical sulcus surgery, 77–78
   keloids, 19–22
Schwalbe, 24
Sculpted costal cartilage, 101. See also Cartilage
Secondary otoplasty, 3–9
Secondary rhinoplasty, 3
Secondary strictures, of reconstructed canal, 99, 100
Second branchial arch, 27
Sensation
   auricle and, 55–56
   in auriculoplasty, 19
Severe microtia. See Bilateral microtia; Microtia
Sideburn, 111, 113
Silicone, 54
Single-tract fistula, 36–37
Skeletal formation, of auricle, 55
Skeletal support, in microtia, 66
Skeletal system, origination of, 28–29
Skeletal tissue, cartilage and, 44
Skin
   conchal, 22
   and cryptotia, 11
Skin color, of auricle, 57
Skin covering, and auricular integument, 68–69

Skin flaps, 39–40, 67–68. *See also* Grafting; Skin grafts
  in reconstructive ear surgery, 15–17
Skin function, of auricle, 56–57
Skin grafts, 39, 40–41. *See also* Grafting; Skin flaps
  covering neotympanic membrane, 94–98
  and helical sulcus, 74
  inguinal, 105
  from prepuce, 95
  to surround ear, 111
  thick and thin, 94–95
Skull fixation, 90–91
SMAS
  auricular, 86
  auricular integument and, 70–71
  contracture test, 105
  correction, 10
  microtia and repair of, 72
  tropic SMAS, 29
Smoking, during postoperative period, 17
Snail shell ear, 59
Soft tissue repair, in hemifacial microsomia, 66
Somatic period, 28
Somites, 29
Sound reception, 55
Stapedial artery, 28
Stereotactic surgery, 89–94
  for congenital microtia and atresia, 97
Streeter, 24
Strictures, secondary, 99
Strontium 90, beta therapy with, 22
Subtotal avulsion, of auricle, 14
Sulcus, helical, 72–86
Superficial canal, 35
Suppuration, in otitis media, 33–34
Supranumerary tympanic bones, 87
Surgery. *See also* Instruments
  aesthetic, 66
  auricle and, 58
  covering neotympanic membrane, 94–98
  for deficient tragus, 83
  meatomyringoplasty, 88–89, 98–99
  microsurgery, 115
  for partial auricular atresia syndromes, 36
  plastic, 66
  stereotactic, 89–94
Surgical procedure
  for correcting cryptotia and satyr ear, 11–13
  for correcting deformed ears, 5–7
  helical sulcus sequence, 73–80
  for posttraumatic keloid pathology, 20–22
  for repairing traumatic ear loss, 15–19
  for unilateral microtia and atresia, 32–33, 37–42
Suturing, after helical sulcus surgery, 85
Synchronic action, of frontalis and auricularis superioris muscles, 10
Syndromes. *See* syndromes by name

—t—
Tanzer, Radford, 114, 115
Techniques, for ear surgery, 115
Temporomandibular (TM) joint, 14, 19, 88
Therapy
  beta therapy, 22
  neuroendocrine medication and, 22
Thick skin grafts, 94
Thin skin grafts, 94
Tissue
  cartilage and, 44
  delicacy of, 23
TMJ. *See* Temporomandibular (TM) joint
Total atresia, 111–114
  auricular, 86–87
  and partial atresia, 35
Total canal repair, results of, 98–99
Tragus, 35–36, 67–68
  absent, 84
  canoe ear and, 63
  deficient, 83
Transillumination, to measure delicacy of ear, 23
Trauma, otoplasty for, 13–19
Trophic organ, auricle as, 56
Trophic SMAS, 29
Tubotympanic pouch syndrome, 66
"Tunnel" method, 17
Tympanic atresic bone, 91
Tympanic bone, 41–42, 87
Tympanic membrane, layers of, 30
Tympanic ossification, 87
Tympanic pouch, 30
Tympanic ring, 29–31, 87

—u—
Undermining, 6
Unilateral atresia, 32–33
  case study of, 37–42
  wisdom of operating on, 33–34
Unilateral microtia. *See also* Microtia
  case study of, 37–42
  donor ear and, 67
  tragus and, 67–68
  wisdom of operating on, 33–34
Upper nubbin, and bilateral atresia, 104

—v—
Vertical measures, and otoplasty, 7, 8
Viscera, auricle as, 70

—w—
Waldeyer's circle, 27
White fibrocartilage, 44

—y—
Yellow elastic cartilage, 44

—z—
Z-plasty
  auricular integument and, 69
  unilateral microtia and, 68

MIX
Papier aus verantwortungsvollen Quellen
Paper from responsible sources
FSC® C105338

If you have any concerns about our products,
you can contact us on
ProductSafety@springernature.com

In case Publisher is established outside the EU,
the EU authorized representative is:
**Springer Nature Customer Service Center GmbH
Europaplatz 3, 69115 Heidelberg, Germany**

Printed by Libri Plureos GmbH
in Hamburg, Germany